OFFICE OF POPULATION CENSUSES AND S
SOCIAL SURVEY DIVISION

Infant feeding 1985

A survey carried out by Social Survey Division of OPCS on behalf of the Department of Health and Social Security and the Scottish Home and Health Department

Jean Martin

Amanda White

MEDICAL LIBRARY
WATFORD POSTGRADUATE
MEDICAL CENTRE
WATFORD GENERAL HOSPITAL
VICARAGE ROAD
WATFORD WD1 8HB

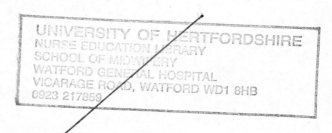

UNIVERSITY OF HERTFORDSHIRE
NURSE EDUCATION LIBRARY
SCHOOL OF MIDWIFERY
WATFORD GENERAL HOSPITAL
VICARAGE ROAD, WATFORD WD1 8HB
0923 217859

WEST HERTFORDSHIRE
SCHOOL OF MIDWIFERY

London: Her Majesty's Stationery Office

© Crown copyright 1988
First published 1988

ISBN 011 691227 8

Her Majesty's Stationery Office

Standing order service

Placing a standing order with HMSO BOOKS enables a customer to receive future editions of this title automatically as published.
This saves the time, trouble and expense of placing individual orders and avoids the problem of knowing when to do so.
For details please write to HMSO BOOKS (PC 13A/1), Publications Centre, PO Box 276, London SW8 5DT and quoting reference X25 08 06.
The standing order service also enables customers to receive automatically as published all material of their choice which additionally saves extensive catalogue research. The scope and selectivity of the service has been extended by new techniques, and there are more than 3,500 classifications to choose from. A special leaflet describing the service in detail may be obtained on request.

Acknowledgements

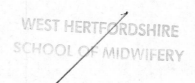

WEST HERTFORDSHIRE
SCHOOL OF MIDWIFERY

We would like to thank everybody who helped to make this survey possible. First of all, the other staff at Social Survey Division who contributed to the different stages of the survey, in particular to Ms L Dowds. We would also like to thank staff in Vital Statistics Branch at OPCS and the GRO in Scotland who drew the sample for us. We are grateful to the Working Party of the Panel on Child Nutrition for its valuable advice and criticism, and in particular to Professor T E Oppé for his encouragement and support throughout the project. Finally we would like to thank the mothers who participated in the project, without whose co-operation the survey would not have been possible.

Front cover shows the National Baby Care symbol.

Contents

List of tables

List of figures

Notes on the tables

Base numbers have been given in italics. Where a base number is less than 30, percentages have not been given but the actual number of cases is shown. Percentages of less than one per cent are shown as 0; cells with no cases are indicated by –.

The varying positions of percentage signs and bases in the tables denote the presentation of different types of information. Where there is a percentage sign at the head of a column and the base at the foot the whole distribution is presented and the figures add up to 100%. Where there is no percentage sign in the table and a note in italics above the figures, the figures refer to the proportion of people who had the attribute being discussed and the complementary proportion (not shown in the table) did not. In the more complex tables both the side and column headings define the group under discussion, the percentage indicating the proportion of the group who have a particular attribute.

Details of significance tests are not given in the report, but they have been carried out where appropriate. Differences referred to in the text are significant at the .05 level.

The term 'bottle fed' as used in this report refers to infants receiving infant formula. Some of the infants, particularly when they were older, would have been receiving infant formula from a lidded cup rather than a bottle.

Symbols used:
.. Not available
0 Denotes less than 0.5%
– Denotes no cases

Summary of main findings and conclusions

Incidence and duration of breast feeding (Chapter 2)

Trends in the incidence of breast feeding (2.1)

There has been no significant change in the incidence of breast feeding in Great Britain between 1980 and 1985. In 1985, 64% of mothers breast fed initially compared with 65% in 1980. This picture of no change was also true in England and Wales and in Scotland separately, and suggests that the increase noted in England and Wales between 1975 and 1980 has stopped.

This overall picture of no change since 1980 did not occur in all subgroups of mothers examined. In particular among mothers of first babies the incidence of breast feeding fell from 74% in 1980 to 69% in 1985. There was also a substantial fall in the incidence of breast feeding among mothers with no partner or whose partner's social class could not be classified (from 52% to 44%) and among mothers of first babies who left school at 16 or under (from 65% to 58%).

Factors associated with the incidence of breast feeding (2.1.1–2.1.9)

As the previous surveys showed the highest incidence of breast feeding was found among mothers of first babies (particularly those who had their first baby when aged over 25), those in the higher social classes, those who were educated beyond the age of 18 and those living in London and the South East.

Whether or not a mother breast fed a second or subsequent child was strongly related to the length of time she had breast fed her first child; the longer she had done so the more likely she was to breast feed again.

In 1985 there was no evidence to show that mothers who were working six weeks after the birth were any less likely to begin breast feeding than mothers who were not working. Mothers who were on maternity leave had the highest incidence of breast feeding, probably a reflection of their higher social class.

Women who smoked, either before or during pregnancy, were considerably less likely to have started breast feeding than those who did not smoke; 46% compared with 71%. Part of the difference was accounted for by the relationship between smoking and social class, but smokers were less likely than non-smokers to breast feed in each of the social class groups.

The overall decrease in breast feeding among mothers of first babies is of concern. This survey and the two previous ones have shown clearly that whether or not a mother breast feeds a second or subsequent baby de-pends mainly on her experience of feeding her first. Few mothers who have chosen not to breast feed their first baby will reverse the decision with subsequent children. The decrease in the incidence of breast feeding since 1980 among mothers of first babies is likely to lead to a decrease in breast feeding among mothers of second and later babies in subsequent years.

Prevalence of breast feeding (2.2)

Overall in Great Britain there has been virtually no change between 1980 and 1985 in the prevalence of breast feeding at ages up to nine months. The separate rates for England and Wales and for Scotland also show very little change over this period. Only 26% of mothers in Great Britain as a whole were still breast feeding at four months.

Trends in the duration of breast feeding (2.3)

The length of time for which mothers who breast fed continued to do so also showed little change between 1980 and 1985. This was true for Great Britain as a whole and for England and Wales and Scotland separately. This lack of change in the duration of breast feeding compared with 1980 occurred in all the subgroups examined. Over one third of mothers who started breast feeding in 1985 stopped within six weeks and only two fifths continued for as long as four months.

Factors associated with the duration of breast feeding (2.3.1–2.3.9)

Mothers who were most likely to have still been breast feeding at six weeks were those with previous experience of breast feeding, those in the higher social classes, those educated beyond the age of 18, those living in the south of England, and those who were non-smokers. The 1985 survey found no evidence that returning to work significantly shortened the length of time for which a mother continued to breast feed.

The latest survey results show that the recommendation in Present day practice in infant feeding, 1980[4] that 'mothers should breast feed their babies, preferably for four to six months, but at least for the first few weeks of life' was nowhere near being achieved. Only 51% of mothers in Great Britain breast fed even for as long as two weeks and only 26% breast fed for four months or more.

In view of the lack of increase in breast feeding since 1980 one might think that the taking up of breast feeding has reached saturation point. This may be the case among mothers in the highest social class groups but given the marked social class gradient in both the incidence and the duration of breast feeding there seems to be scope for encouraging more mothers to breast feed. *Present day practice in infant feeding: third report*[5] recommends 'the search for new ways of encouraging breast feeding especially in those sections of the community where it is shown to be low.' It is particularly important that mothers who have no husband or partner are encouraged to breast feed as it was among this group that the lowest rates of breast feeding were observed. Clearly these mothers will require advice and support so that they can breast feed successfully.

Influences on choice of method of feeding (Chapter 3)

Choice of method of feeding (3.2)
Most women (94%) had decided before the birth on their method of feeding; 61% planned to breast feed and 33% to bottle feed – similar proportions to the 1980 figures. As in 1980, the majority of mothers (95%) carried out their intentions. Previous experience of breast feeding had a strong influence on whether mothers of second or subsequent babies planned to breast feed again.

The reasons given by mothers for planning to breast or bottle feed were very similar to those given in 1980. By far the most common reason given for choosing to breast feed was that breast feeding was thought to be best for the baby, but the convenience of breast feeding was also mentioned by many mothers. Those who chose bottle feeding most frequently mentioned the fact that other people could feed the baby (mothers of first births) or their own previous experience (mothers of later births). Mothers of first babies who chose to bottle feed were particularly likely to say that they did not like the idea of breast feeding.

Contact with health professionals during the antenatal period (3.3)
Almost all mothers in the survey (99%) received antenatal care. Although 88% said they had been asked how they intended to feed their baby at antenatal checkups it is still noteworthy that 12% said that they had not; this was however an improvement on the 1980 figure of 16%. There were only 41% of mothers who said they had been both asked about their plans for feeding the baby and had a discussion – not significantly different from the 1980 figure of 39%. However among women having their first baby the figure was higher – 49%; a significant increase on the 1980 figure of 45%.

Antenatal classes were attended mainly by women expecting first babies and since 1980 there has been a significant increase in the proportion attending, 71% compared with 67%. As in 1980 the majority of mothers of first babies who attended classes said that they included talks or discussions about feeding babies (86%); 83% said that they had been told about the advantages of breast feeding and 59% that they had been taught how to make up a bottle.

As in 1980 attendance at antenatal classes was associated with a higher than average likelihood of planning to breast feed. This was true among women in each of the social class groups. This does not necessarily imply a causal relationship as women who were already planning to breast feed might be more likely to attend classes anyway.

In 1985, 56% of mothers had been visited by a midwife or health visitor at home during their pregnancy, a significant increase on the 53% who had received such a visit in 1980. In 1985 such visits did show a relationship with planning to breast feed, those receiving a visit being more likely to be planning to breast feed than those who did not. No such relationship had been found in 1980.

Present day practice in infant feeding: third report[5] recommends that 'all parents have the opportunity for a discussion with an informed person about infant feeding during the antenatal period'. It seems wise to do this at antenatal checkups rather than just at antenatal classes as many women do not attend the classes, particularly those expecting a second or subsequent baby and those in the lower social classes who, as we have seen, are in particular need of help and advice to encourage them to both start and to continue breast feeding successfully.

Literature containing information on feeding babies (3.4)
In 1985 most mothers had received a copy of *The Pregnancy Book* as well as other free books or phamplets containing information about feeding babies. Only 2% of those expecting their first baby and 7% of other mothers said that they had not been given any free literature about feeding babies.

Lessons on parentcraft at school (3.5)
Whether or not mothers had any lessons on parentcraft or child development when they were at school did not appear to be associated with intentions to breast feed.

Influences on the duration of breast feeding (Chapter 4)

Reasons for stopping breast feeding (4.2)
The reasons mothers gave for stopping breast feeding in 1985 were broadly similar to those given in 1980. Insufficient milk was the most frequently given reason. Sore nipples or the baby not sucking properly were reasons given by mothers who stopped breast feeding in the first week or so. Only among mothers who had breast fed for longer than four months was 'breast feeding for as long as intended' the dominant reason.

Factors associated with stopping breast feeding in the early weeks (4.3–4.12)
Despite the decrease since 1980 in the average length of stay in hospital, in 1985 15% of mothers who started breast feeding had given up before they left hospital – the same proportion as in 1980. Since altogether 19% gave up in the first two weeks, only 4% gave up in the remainder of the first two weeks following discharge. These results do not support the view that women manage to breast feed while in hospital only to stop when

they get home where less help is available. The steepest drop in the prevalence of breast feeding occurs in the first week of life, so the period in hospital is particularly important.

As had been the case in the previous surveys a number of events occurring around the time of the birth and various hospital practices were found to be associated with the probability of stopping breast feeding in the first two weeks.

Mothers who experienced particular problems around the time of the birth were the most likely to stop breast feeding in the first two weeks. Having a caesarian delivery, particularly one under a general anaesthetic, having a baby who had to go into special care or having a low birthweight baby were all associated with the early cessation of breast feeding. Mothers who first put their baby to the breast more than an hour after the birth were also likely to stop breast feeding early. Further analysis showed that of these factors delays in starting breast feeding had the most effect on stopping breast feeding in the first two weeks. Even if mothers did not have any of the other problems mentioned above they were still more likely to stop breast feeding in the first two weeks if they put their baby to the breast more than an hour after the birth than if they initiated breast feeding sooner. The other factors only affected the likelihood of stopping breast feeding by virtue of their association with delays in starting breast feeding.

This survey showed that changes in hospital practices had occurred since the earlier surveys. The proportion of mothers reporting that they had to feed at set times had declined significantly between 1975 and 1980. By 1985 there had been a further decline; only 19% of breast feeding mothers reported having to feed at set times compared with 32% in 1980. Mothers were more likely to have their babies with them for most of their stay in hospital in 1985 than they had been in 1980; 47% said their baby was with them continuously compared with only 17% in 1980. Mothers were initiating breast feeding sooner after the birth. In 1985, 27% had put their baby to the breast immediately compared with only 16% in 1980. However, there was very little change since 1980 in the proportion of breast fed babies who had been given bottles of infant formula while in hospital: in 1985 almost half of the mothers reported that their baby had received some in the first week of life.

Giving infant formula in the first week was associated with stopping breast feeding within two weeks. Other hospital practices which were found to be associated with the cessation of breast feeding were the hospital feeding routine and how soon the baby was first put to the breast. Of these, whether or not the baby had been given infant formula in the first week had the most effect.

Despite the changes in hospital practices mentioned above, this did not result in fewer mothers stopping breast feeding within the first two weeks.

Present day practice in infant feeding: third report[5] recommends that 'those responsible for the care of the mother who intends to breast feed and her baby encourage the practices associated with successful initiation of breast feeding including early breast feeding after birth, on-demand feeding, "rooming-in" of mothers and babies, and the avoidance of complementary feeds or fluids of any sort'.

Problems with breast feeding in the early weeks (4.13 and 4.14)
In 1985, 30% of breast feeding mothers reported having feeding problems while still in hospital. Sore or cracked nipples was the most common problem experienced. The vast majority of breast feeding mothers said that they were able to get help or advice in hospital when they needed it; only 5% said this was not the case.

Of those who were breast feeding at all when they left hospital 30% had given up by six weeks. Those most likely to have given up by six weeks were those who were giving both breast and bottle when they left hospital, those who kept to set feeding schedules rather than feeding on demand and those who experienced feeding problems once they had returned home. The most common feeding problem reported by breast feeding mothers at this stage was that the baby was hungry – presumably they meant the baby was crying with what appeared to be hunger. As professional advice is not always available it is important that mothers are forewarned of the common problems with breast feeding in the early weeks and how they may be prevented or overcome without the mother having to give up breast feeding.

Infant formula and bottle feeding (Chapter 5)

The prevalence of bottle feeding (5.1)
Although in 1985 the majority of mothers started breast feeding, 36% gave infant formula feeds from birth. Of those who started breast feeding 39% had stopped by six weeks and some of those who continued were giving formula as well as breast feeds. Thus by the time they were six weeks old 62% of babies in Great Britain were being fed infant formulas and at four months three quarters of babies were fully bottle fed. In 1985 breast fed babies were more likely to be receiving bottles in addition to breast milk than had been the case in 1980. Thus although there was little change in either the incidence or the duration of breast feeding between 1980 and 1985, it appears that bottle feeding was more widespread in 1985 as more breast fed babies were also being given bottle feeds.

Advice about bottle feeding (5.5 and 5.7)
Most mothers expecting their first baby who attended antenatal classes reported being shown how to make up a bottle (59%) – 41% said that they had not been shown. Mothers who intended to bottle feed were no more likely to have been shown than those who intended to breast feed.

Given that many mothers are bottle feeding *Present day practice in infant feeding: third report*[5] recommends that 'parents receive advice about infant formulas and about the preparation of feeds'.

The most common feeding problem experienced by bottle feeding mothers once they had left hospital was that the baby appeared to be hungry – as was the case with breast feeders. Thus all mothers need to be forewarned that this is a very common problem and given advice on what they might do so that they are more able to cope with it.

Free samples of infant formula (5.6)
A quarter of those mothers who were giving only breast milk on discharge from hospital said they were given a free sample of infant formula to take home. This practice is not in conformity with the WHO code and may be associated with a premature resort to artificial feeding. However, there was no evidence from this survey that these mothers stopped breast feeding any sooner than those who did not receive a free sample of infant formula. *Present day practice in infant feeding: third report*[5] recommends that 'samples of infant formula should not be given to mothers'.

The use of non-human milk at different ages (5.4)
The main type of non-human milk given to babies varied with the baby's age. At birth and when the baby was about six weeks old whey dominant infant formula was the predominant non-human milk given. Once the baby was about four months old casein dominant formula had become the predominant non-human milk. When the baby had reached about nine months old liquid cow's milk had taken over as the main milk. Although it is not recommended that liquid cow's milk should be used as the main milk in the diet of very young infants it can form part of the diet of older infants. The survey found that in most cases it was not until the baby was over six months old that liquid cow's milk had been introduced. Only 4% of mothers had given liquid cow's milk as the main drink before five months, and the majority had not done so until the baby was at least six months old. Very few mothers used 'follow-up milks' at any stage, only 1% were giving them when the baby was aged nine months.

The pattern of milk usage followed by mothers who were bottle feeding exclusively was broadly similar to that followed by mothers who were breast feeding as well, the main differences being that those who were breast feeding as well were more likely to be giving a whey dominant formula at six weeks and were more likely to be giving liquid cow's milk at four months and at nine months.

Solid food, vitamins and other drinks (Chapter 6)

Trends in feeding practices (6.2)
There has not been a great deal of change since 1980 in the age at which mothers introduced solid foods. This is in contrast to the major change observed between 1975 and 1980 when the proportion of mothers giving solids

before three months had fallen sharply from 85% to 56%. In 1985 the figure was 62%. As in 1975 and in 1980, the 1985 survey found that mothers who were bottle feeding tended to introduce solids earlier than those who were breast feeding. Possibly such mothers are reluctant to increase the amount of milk given in response to the baby's hunger and give solids instead. Mothers most likely to have introduced solids by three months were those in the lower social classes, those living in Scotland and the North of England and those who smoked.

Present day practice in infant feeding: third report[5] states that 'few infants will require solid foods before the age of three months but the majority should be offered a mixed diet not later than the age of six months', however as stated above almost two thirds of babies had received solids by three months.

Solid foods given at different ages (6.3)
In 1985 cereals and rusks were still the most common first solid foods as they had been in 1975 and 1980. By about four months the majority of mothers (90%) were giving solids and many babies were eating commercial babyfood. When asked what factors they took into account when deciding what solid foods to give 'general nutrition' was the factor mothers mentioned most frequently. Other considerations were the sugar content of the food and the variety of foods. Sugar was the ingredient most often avoided by mothers, the reason often given was that it was not good for the baby and that it was bad for developing teeth.

Additional drinks (6.5)
The proportion of breast fed babies who were receiving additional drinks at six weeks was lower in 1985 than it had been in 1980; 68% compared with 76%. However among bottle fed babies there was no change. In 1985 bottle fed babies were more likely than those who were breast fed to have been given additional drinks at this age, this had also been the case in 1980. At this age the majority of those giving drinks were giving plain water but considerable numbers of mothers were giving sweetened baby drinks, for example 34% were giving baby drinks sweetened with sugar or glucose.

Present day practice in infant feeding: third report[5] states that there is some doubt about the need for young babies to receive drinks in addition to breast milk or infant formula. Although there is a range of products designed to add flavouring to water (the flavours may be herbal such as fennel or vanilla or based on fruit juices) many of these also contain sugar. Thirsty infants will take water without sugar or flavouring, there is no need to give them sweetened drinks.

Supplementary vitamins (6.6)
Young infants who are being breast fed or given infant formula are unlikely to become vitamin deficient. Since 1980 there has been a considerable fall in the proportion of babies receiving supplementary vitamins. In 1985, 35% of mothers were giving supplementary vita-

mins at four months compared with 47% in 1980. This in itself is not alarming as the majority of babies of this age in 1985 were receiving infant formula, which is fortified with the necessary vitamins. However, as the contribution from these milks to the overall mixed diet declines, and as the vitamin stores wane, supplementary vitamins are recommended. Of babies at nine months who were receiving no breast or formula milks, only 45% were being given vitamin drops.

To guard against any infants becoming vitamin deficient *Present day practice in infant feeding: third report*[5] recommends that 'vitamin supplementation should be given to infants and young children aged from six months up to at least two years and preferably five years.'

Problems with feeding and changing (6.7 and 6.8)
Although the proportion of mothers who reported having feeding problems declined as the babies got older (22% at four months and 15% at nine months), problems with giving solids were mentioned increasingly by those mothers who did have problems. Of those who had problems at four months 11% said the baby would not take solids and at nine months 29% said their baby would only take certain solids.

The 1985 survey found that most mothers would welcome more facilities in public places for feeding and for changing babies. *Present day practice in infant feeding: third report*[5] is 'concerned that breast feeding has not yet gained complete social acceptance as the usual way of feeding babies. We urge social, community, educational, commercial and other concerns to take a positive approach to this matter.'

Conclusion
The results of this survey have shown that the increases in the incidence and the duration of breast feeding seen between 1975 and 1980 have not continued up until 1985. The picture of infant feeding observed in 1985 was in many ways very similar to that in 1980, with no significant changes in either the incidence or the duration of breast feeding. However, there was a decrease in both the proportion of mothers attempting to breast feed and the length of time for which they continued to do so among mothers of first babies who had no husband or partner. A significant minority of mothers were still choosing not to breast feed in 1985 and, more importantly, many mothers who began breast feeding did not manage to do so for more than a few weeks. As the Health Departments in England and Wales and in Scotland consider it is important to continue the monitoring of infant feeding practice as recommended by the original Working Party of the Panel of Child Nutrition it is planned that OPCS will conduct a further survey in 1990.

1 Introduction

1.1 Background to the survey
This is the third survey of infant feeding carried out by the Office of Population Censuses and Surveys on behalf of the Department of Health and Social Security. The surveys were commissioned in response to the recommendation of the Committee on Medical Aspects of Food Policy (COMA) that provisions should be made for a 'continuous review of patterns of infant feeding'. The first survey took place in 1975[1] and provided baseline statistics about infant feeding practices in England and Wales. The second and third surveys, in 1980[2] and 1985 also covered Scotland and have examined changes since 1975.

In 1974 the Panel on Child Nutrition, which is a subcommittee of COMA set up a Working Party to review current practices in feeding normal infants and their effects on infants' well-being[3]. It concluded that all mothers should be encouraged to breast feed their babies, preferably for four to six months, but at least for the first few weeks of life. It also concluded that the introduction of solids before about four months should be discouraged.

Since this first report in 1974 there have been two further reports on infant feeding from COMA, in 1980[4] and 1988[5]. Both recommended that regular surveys should continue at intervals of approximately five years and they endorsed the earlier recommendations.

1.2 Aims of the 1985 survey
Although there are common aims to all three surveys, each has some individual aims and the 1985 survey also covers some new topics not included in the previous surveys. Its main aims are:

(a) to establish how mothers feed their infants and what changes have occurred since 1980

(b) to investigate changes in infant feeding in the early weeks and the factors associated with these changes

(c) to establish the age at which solid foods are introduced and to examine weaning practices up to nine months.

1.3 Definitions used in the survey
A number of terms defined for the 1975 and 1980 surveys are used throughout this report. The definitions are as follows:

Breast fed initially refers to all babies whose mothers put them to the breast at all, even if this was on one occasion only.

Incidence of breast feeding is the proportion of sampled babies who were breast fed initially.

Still breast fed refers to all babies whose mothers were breast feeding at all at a specified age, even if they were also bottle fed or receiving other food.

Prevalence of breast feeding refers to the proportion of all sampled babies still being wholly or partially breast fed at specified ages.

Duration of breast feeding is the length of time for which breast feeding continued at all, regardless of when bottles or foods other than milk were introduced.

1.4 Design of the 1985 survey
An important factor governing the design of the 1985 survey was the need to be able to make comparisons with the previous surveys. Therefore the basic design was the same as for the 1980 survey. However, three changes were made:

(i) *A larger sample of mothers was selected initially*
This was done partly because it was expected that changes in breast feeding would be decreasing over time and so larger numbers would be required to detect significant changes in the subgroups of interest. This does not affect comparisons between 1980 and 1985 because the precision of the estimates of change is constrained by the smaller of the two samples, but it will be important for future comparisons.

Secondly, a larger sample allows more detailed examination of particular subgroups before the size of the group becomes too small for meaningful percentages to be calculated.

(ii) *Mothers in Social Class V and mothers whose social class was unclassified were oversampled*
Both the previous surveys had established strong associations between social class and various infant feeding practices: in general mothers in the lower social classes or with least formal education were those least likely to conform to the DHSS recommendations for good practice. The previous two surveys had established that these mothers had the lowest rates of breast feeding and those that started breast feeding gave up soonest. They were also particularly likely to start giving their babies solid foods earlier than other mothers. Since they form rather small groups in a random sample of mothers it was decided to give them twice the chance of selection compared with other mothers. In all the analyses presented in this report the results for these mothers have been downweighted by a factor of two to

allow for this oversampling before they are added to results for other mothers. However, results can often be shown separately for these groups since their true numbers are greater than the reweighted base numbers.

(iii) *All mothers were followed up until nine months*
The previous two surveys had paid particular attention to feeding in the first half of infancy and while this information was still required, it was felt that the 1985 survey should collect more detailed information about later infancy. This led to the decision to ask more detailed questions about weaning foods and to follow up all mothers until their babies were at least nine months old, rather than just those who were breast feeding at the previous contact, as had been done on the other two surveys.

The main features of the sample design of the 1985 survey are described in the following section.

1.5 Sample design
The sample was designed to be representative of births occurring in England and Wales between 17 August and 13 September 1985 which had been registered within four weeks of the birth. In Scotland the sample was of births occurring between 10 August and 20 September which had been registered within three weeks of the birth.

The sampling frame for England and Wales consisted of the draft birth registrations received by Vital Statistics Branch of OPCS. A sample of 100 registration sub-districts, grouped as necessary, was selected. As far as possible these were the same sub-districts as used on the 1980 survey, but changes in the birth rates in a number of sub-districts necessitated some changes.

Within the selected sub-districts a systematic random sample of births was selected. Social class was coded on the basis of the information about the father's occupation recorded on the draft birth registration. The coding procedures normally used by Vital Statistics Branch were applied. All births coded as Social Class V or which were in the 'unclassified' category (mainly because the mother had no known partner) were selected for the survey. One in two of all other births were selected. Thus 5,805 births in all were selected for the survey in England and Wales.

In Scotland birth registrations are received by the General Registrar Office (Scotland) and put onto computer within one week. This meant that computer rather than manual procedures could be used. Social class had already been coded and was shown on the computer print-out. It was therefore a simple matter to carry out the same procedure of rejecting every one in two births coded to Social Classes I to IV as had been done in England and Wales. In Scotland a total of 2,349 births were selected.

Thus a total of 8,154 births were selected in Great Britain.

1.6 Procedure
For the first stage questionnaires were sent out during September and October 1985 to mothers of 8,154 babies born within the appropriate weeks. Those failing to reply after two weeks were sent a reminder letter and a second reminder was sent after a further two weeks if necessary. Interviewers were sent to contact mothers who had failed to reply after two reminder letters.

In January 1986 (when the babies were at least four months old) second stage questionnaires were sent to the 7,390 mothers who had completed the first questionnaire. In June 1986 (when the babies were at least nine months old) third stage questionnaires were sent to all those 5,958 mothers who had completed the second stage questionnaire. At both the second and third stages a small number of mothers were not contacted because although they had completed the previous stage they asked not to be contacted again.

1.7 Response
At the first stage a sample of 8,154 babies was selected and the mothers approached by post. Those who failed to respond, even after two reminders, were contacted by interviewer. The overall response rate was 91%. Table 1.1 summarises the losses due to various sources of non-response.

Mothers were not asked to complete a questionnaire if they were separated from their baby for any reason (for instance if the baby had died, been adopted, or was in hospital). Such mothers were asked to indicate this on the front of the questionnaire and then to return the blank questionnaire so they would not be troubled again. Included in 'refusal' are those who returned a

Table 1.1 Response rates and non-response at the first stage (six weeks or more)

	England and Wales		Scotland		Great Britain	
	No	%	No	%	No	%
Initial sample	5,805	100	2,349	100	8,154	100
Total response	**5,273**	**91**	**2,123**	**90**	**7,396**	**91**
due to postal enquiry	4,773	82	1,951	83	6,724	83
due to interviewer contact	500	9	172	7	672	8
Total non-response	**532**	**9**	**226**	**10**	**758**	**9**
baby not with mother	46	1	17	1	63	1
refusal	99	2	22	1	121	1
post returned/not delivered	82	1	48	2	130	2
no reply from postal stage and interviewer unable to contact	305	5	139	6	444	5

Table 1.2 Response rates and non-response at the second stage (four months or more)

	England and Wales		Scotland		Great Britain	
	No	%	No	%	No	%
Second stage sample	5,273	100	2,123	100	7,396	100
Total response	**4,260**	**81**	**1,709**	**81**	**5,969**	**81**
Total non-response	**1,013**	**19**	**414**	**19**	**1,427**	**19**
refused at first stage	4	0	2	0	6	0
baby not with mother	17	0	8	0	25	0
refusal	35	1	9	0	44	1
post returned/not delivered	75	1	47	2	122	2
no reply	882	17	348	16	1,230	17

Table 1.3 Response rates and non-response at the third stage (nine months or more)

	England and Wales		Scotland		Great Britain	
	No	%	No	%	No	%
Third stage sample	4,260	100	1,709	100	5,969	100
Total response	**3,532**	**83**	**1,414**	**83**	**4,946**	**83**
Total non-response	**728**	**17**	**295**	**17**	**1,023**	**17**
refused at second stage	10	0	1	0	11	0
baby not with mother	6	0	8	0	14	0
refusal	8	0	3	0	11	0
post returned/not delivered	71	2	60	4	131	2
no reply	633	15	223	13	856	14

Table 1.4 Summary of response at the three stages

	England and Wales		Scotland		Great Britain	
	No	%	No	%	No	%
Initial sample	5,805	100	2,349	100	8,154	100
Response at stage 1	5,273	91	2,123	90	7,396	91
Response at stage 2	4,260	73	1,709	73	5,969	73
Response at stage 3	3,532	61	1,414	60	4,946	61

blank questionnaire with no explanation, as well as those explicitly refusing to co-operate. 'Post returned/ not delivered' includes both questionnaires returned by the Post Office and those returned by someone other than the mother saying that she no longer lived at the address to which we had written. Wherever possible questionnaires were sent to any forwarding address given to us and every effort was made to provide a more detailed address where the Post Office required it in order to deliver the envelope.

At the second stage 7,390 mothers were written to again and a response rate of 81% was obtained. Details of the non-response are given in Table 1.2

5,958 mothers were written to at the final stage and 83% responded. Table 1.3 shows the details of the non-response.

Since at the second and third stages only mothers who had responded at the previous stage were contacted, the effect of non-response at each stage is cumulative. Table 1.4 shows the response at each stage as a proportion of the initial sample. Thus at the second stage

questionnaires were received from 73% of the original sample, while by the third stage this proportion had fallen to 61%.

1.8 Reweighting the results

In order to obtain a sufficiently large sample of births in Scotland for separate analysis, births in Scotland were given a greater chance of selection than those in England and Wales. So that results for Scotland could be added in their correct proportion to those for England and Wales, the Scottish results were reweighted by a factor of 0.291.

As babies born to mothers in Social Class V or whose social class was unclassifiable had been given twice the chance of selection compared with other babies, the results for these mothers had to be reweighted by a factor of 0.5 to make them comparable with the results of other mothers.

Applying both these reweighting factors to the main stage sample gives a total weighted sample of 5,223 completed questionnaires for Great Britain, made up of 4,671 questionnaires for England and Wales and 552 questionnaires for Scotland.

Data obtained from the second and third stage questionnaires required additional reweighting to adjust for the non-response to each of these stages. The reweighting factors were calculated to take account of the differing levels of response obtained from mothers in different social class groups and to arrive at the same weighted sample as at the first stage questionnaire (5,223). This was done to facilitate comparisons between different tables and parts of tables. However calculations of sampling errors and tests of significance have been based on the actual number of questionnaires rather than on the weighted totals shown in the tables. All tables displaying data from the second and third stages include percentages based on a smaller number of individuals than is suggested by the weighted base presented. These tables have been marked to draw attention to the fact that such percentages are subject to larger errors than those based on data at the first stage.

1.9 Making comparisons with the 1980 results

One of the main purposes of the 1985 survey was to provide data to establish trends in infant feeding. There are several factors affecting comparisons made over time and before we present the results it is important to consider their effect on the interpretation of the data. Firstly, sample size is a major determinant of the capacity to measure change. Because of this, the sample was designed to be sufficiently large for comparisons to be made for the important subgroups.

Secondly, it must be remembered that each survey was based on an independent random sample of individuals. Thus the two sets of results are each subject to sampling error and this becomes particularly important when the data are presented for small subgroups. When sampling errors are taken into account an apparent change with time may be seen to be not statistically significant.

Thirdly, both surveys are subject to possible biases due to non-response. Sampling from draft birth registrations meant, however, that a certain amount of information was available about the babies whose mothers did not take part in the survey. Details of the sample validation carried out will be found in Appendix I.

Fourthly, any significant differences between the composition of the 1980 sample and the 1985 sample will affect the comparison over time. Details of the composition of each of the samples is given in Appendix I. On the whole the two samples had very similar characteristics, the only exception being with regard to social class. Table 1.5 shows the distribution of the total sample by social class and separately for mothers of first births and of later births; it also compares the distribution of the two samples with that of the population as a whole in 1980 and 1985. Although for the 1980 sample figures were not shown separately for women whose husband's occupation could not be classified and those with no husband or partner, there has been an overall increase in these two groups combined, from 8% of the total sample in 1980 to 15% in 1985. This increase occurred both among mothers of first births and among mothers of later births and is largely due to the increase since 1980 in the proportion of mothers with no husband or partner. Thus when making comparisons between 1980 and 1985 the increased proportion of this group should be borne in mind.

The observed difference between our two samples is in line with the pattern shown by other available statistics. Between 1980 and 1985 data from birth registrations show that the proportion of illegitimate births in Great Britain increased from 12% to 19% (Table 1.5). In 1985, however, 65% of illegitimate births were registered by both parents which suggests that at least half

Table 1.5 Distribution of the population and the sample by social class for first and later births (1980 and 1985 Great Britain)

Social class of husband/partner	Surveys						Population*	
	First births		Later births		All births			
	1980	1985	1980	1985	1980	1985	1980	1985
	%	%	%	%	%	%	%	%
I & II	25	25	28	26	26	26	25	24
IIINM	10	9	7	8	8	8	10	9
All non-manual	35	34	35	34	34	34	35	33
IIIM	40	30	43	33	42	32	32	28
IV & V	15	16	16	21	16	19	18	16
All manual	55	46	59	54	58	51	50	44
Unclassified	}10	3}20	}6	4}12	}8	4}15	3	4
No husband/partner		16		7		11	..	..
Illegitimate†	..	..	..	..	..	..	12	19
	100	100	100	100	100	100	100	100
Base:	1,831	2,347	2,377	2,875	4,224	5,223	725,000	723,100

* Figures based on live births in Great Britain in 1985
† Births to unmarried mothers

the children born outside marriage had parents who were living together. This explains why the proportion of illegitimate births derived from birth registrations is somewhat higher than the proportion of mothers with no husband or partner found in our 1985 sample. Data from the General Household Survey show that throughout the 1970s and early 1980s lone mothers were becoming an increasingly larger proportion of the population. In 1971 they made up 7% of the population of Great Britain, by 1980 this had increased to 10% and in 1985 it had reached 12%.

2 Incidence and duration of breast feeding

2.1 Incidence of breast feeding

As on the previous two surveys incidence of breast feeding is defined as 'the proportion of babies who were breast fed initially'. This includes all babies who were put to the breast at all, even if this was on one occasion only. Although it can be argued that putting a baby to the breast on only one or two occasions does not really constitute breast feeding, this definition has the advantage of being clear cut and avoids the decision about a necessarily arbitrary criterion of a certain number of attempts or a certain length of time as constituting breast feeding. Moreover, this survey, like the previous two, found that very few mothers stop breast feeding after only a few attempts and so the results would be little changed if a more stringent definition were used.

In 1985 the incidence of breast feeding in Great Britain was 64% (Table 2.1 and Figure 2.1). This compares with a figure of 65% in 1980 and does not represent a statistically significant change between the two surveys. In England and Wales there had been a dramatic increase in the incidence of breast feeding between 1975 and 1980, from 51% to 67%, which then levelled to 65% in 1985. Similarly in Scotland the rates changed from 50% in 1980 to 48% in 1985. So the latest results indicate that the increase seen up to 1980 had stopped.

On both previous surveys a number of factors were shown to be strongly associated with rates of breast feeding. We examine whether these relationships persist in 1985 and whether the overall picture of no change since 1980 masks increases in breast feeding in some subgroups and compensating decreases in others.

2.1.1 Incidence of breast feeding and birth order

As the previous surveys showed, the highest incidence of breast feeding is found among first babies, with successively lower rates for higher birth orders (Table 2.2). Figure 2.2 illustrates the changes between

Table 2.2 **Incidence of breast feeding by birth order (1980 and 1985 Great Britain)**

Birth order	1980	1985	1980	1985
	Percentage who breast fed initially		Bases	
First birth	74	69	1,831	2,347
Second birth	60	60	1,519	1,725
Third birth	56	57	558	737
Fourth or later birth	49	56	281	387
All second and subsequent births*	58	59	2,377	2,875

Includes some babies for whom exact birth order was not known

Figure 2.1 **Incidence of breast feeding by country (1975, 1980 and 1985)**

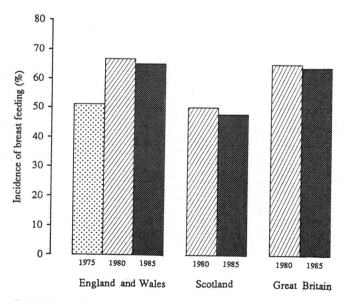

Figure 2.2 **Incidence of breast feeding by birth order (1980 and 1985 Great Britain)**

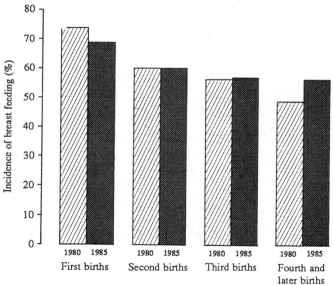

Table 2.1 **Incidence of breast feeding by country (1975, 1980 and 1985)**

	England and Wales			Scotland		Great Britain	
	Percentage who breast fed initially						
	1975	1980	1985	1980	1985	1980	1985
	51	67	65	50	48	65	64
Base:	1,544	3,755	4,671	1,718	1,895	4,224	5,223

6

1980 and 1985 and shows that the decrease in incidence with increasing birth order is less marked in 1985 than it was in 1980. The rates for second and subsequent babies have barely changed – if anything they have risen slightly. But the rate for first babies has fallen from 74% in 1980 to 69% in 1985. This decrease is of concern; the previous surveys showed clearly that whether or not a mother breast feeds a second or subsequent baby depends crucially on her experience of feeding her first. Few mothers who have chosen not to breast feed their first child will reverse the decision with subsequent children. So the rates of breast feeding for second and later babies in 1985 will be determined largely by the experiences of mothers some years ago when their first child was born. The lower rate among mothers of first babies is likely to herald a decrease in breast feeding among these mothers in subsequent years.

2.1.2 Incidence of breast feeding and social class
The analyses in Chapter 1 used information from the birth registration details about the father or partner's occupation to assign social class. In analysing the survey results in this and later chapters the information given on the questionnaires has been used as it usually gave more detail. In the questionnaire mothers were asked whether they were married or living with a part-

Figure 2.3 Incidence of breast feeding by social class (1980 and 1985 Great Britain)

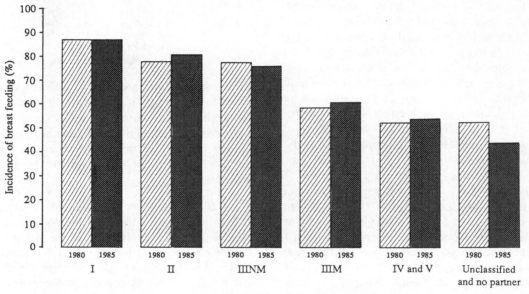

Social class of husband/partner

Table 2.3 Incidence of breast feeding by social class for first and later births (1980 and 1985 Great Britain)

Social class of husband/ partner	First births		Later births		All babies	
	1980	1985	1980	1985	1980	1985
	Percentage who breast fed initially					
I	94	93	83	83	87	87
II	88	87	71	76	78	81
IIINM	89	85	65	68	77	76
All non-manual	90	88	73	75	80	81
IIIM	70	69	52	55	59	61
IV	}64	68 }64	}43	51 }48	}52	58 }54
V		50		38		43
All manual	68	67	50	52	57	58
Unclassified	}51	59 }44	}54	53 }43	}52	55 }44
No partner		41		37		39
All babies	74	69	58	59	65	64
Bases:						
I	*138*	*136*	*196*	*171*	*335*	*307*
II	*311*	*444*	*457*	*584*	*769*	*1,028*
IIINM	*179*	*213*	*175*	*223*	*355*	*436*
All non-manual	*628*	*793*	*828*	*978*	*1,459*	*1,771*
IIIM	*742*	*703*	*1,022*	*962*	*1,769*	*1,666*
IV	}266	*284*	}391	*453*	}659	*738*
V		*103*		*144*		*247*
All manual	*1,009*	*1,090*	*1,413*	*1,559*	*2,428*	*2,651*
Unclassified	}195	*81*	}136	*125*	}336	*207*
No partner		*383*		*212*		*595*
All babies	*1,831*	*2,347*	*2,377*	*2,875*	*4,224*	*5,223*

ner and questions were asked about the partner's occupation enabling social class to be coded.

The social class gradient in breast feeding, with the highest rates among women in the highest social classes, was clearly established in 1975 and is still apparent in 1985. (Table 2.3 and Figure 2.3)

Looking first at the 1985 figures for all births, it can be seen that there is a particularly large difference between Social Class III non-manual (76%) and Social Class III manual (61%), but most striking is the low rate of breast feeding among mothers not living with a husband or partner (39%). Figure 2.3 compares the 1985 figures with those for 1980 and shows that it is among this group that the greatest decrease has taken place. Although in 1980 figures were not shown separately for women whose husband's occupation could not be classified and those with no husband or partner, the overall fall in these two categories combined was from 52% to 44%. Since 1980 there has been a significant increase in the proportion of mothers with no husband or partner, so the breast feeding rate for this group exerts a proportionately greater effect on the overall rate than it did in 1980. There is in fact no evidence of any overall decrease in breast feeding among any of the other social class groups.

Comparing the results for first births separately it can be seen that the overall decrease from 74% in 1980 to 69% in 1985 is accounted for mainly by the significant decrease in breast feeding among mothers with no partner or whose partner's social class was unclassified: 51% to 44%. However there were also small decreases in most of the other social classes. Among the later births a different picture can be seen: most social classes show a slight increase in breast feeding, but this is offset by the substantial decrease among mothers in the unclassified group or with no partner, resulting in no change overall.

2.1.3 Incidence of breast feeding and age at which mother completed full-time education

In 1985, as in 1975 and 1980, mothers who left full-time education at the statutory school-leaving age (16 for most of these women) were least likely to breast feed, while those who had continued in education beyond 18

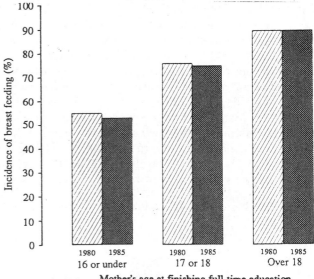

Figure 2.4 Incidence of breast feeding by mother's education (1980 and 1985 Great Britain)

were most likely to do so. Table 2.4 and Figure 2.4 show little change in the overall picture since 1980. However inspection of Table 2.4 shows that although there was no change among mothers of later babies, among mothers of first babies the rate for those who left school at 16 or under fell from 65% to 58%: a significant drop.

2.1.4 Incidence of breast feeding and mothers' age

A mother's age at the birth of second or subsequent children depends on her age at the first birth, the number of children she has had and the spacing between them. It is thus difficult to interpret the significance of any relationship between breast feeding and the age of mothers of second and later babies. For this reason analysis of the effect of mother's age is confined to mothers of first babies (Table 2.5 and Figure 2.5). From the results in the previous two sections a fall in breast feeding since 1980 might be expected among the youngest mothers since they are likely to be in the lowest social classes or not to have a partner, and to have left school at the minimum age. Figure 2.5 shows this to be the case, but also provides evidence of a fall in breast feeding among all mothers who had a first birth when aged under 30; only among those aged 30 or over has there been no change since 1980.

Table 2.4 Incidence of breast feeding by age at which mother completed full-time education and whether first or later births (1980 and 1985 Great Britain)

Age at which mother completed full-time education	First births		Later births		All babies	
	1980	1985	1980	1985	1980	1985
	Percentage who breast fed initially					
16 or under	65	58	48	49	55	53
17 or 18	81	80	70	70	76	75
Over 18	94	94	85	86	89	89
All babies*	74	69	58	59	65	64
Bases:						
16 or under	*1,067*	*1,310*	*1,562*	*1,800*	*2,632*	*3,110*
17 or 18	*453*	*698*	*438*	*648*	*892*	*1,346*
Over 18	*298*	*328*	*358*	*397*	*657*	*725*
*All babies**	*1,831*	*2,347*	*2,377*	*2,875*	*4,224*	*5,223*

* Includes some cases where mother's age at finishing full-time education was not known

Table 2.5 Incidence of breast feeding by mother's age (first births only, 1980 and 1985 Great Britain)

Mother's age	1980	1985	1980	1985
	Percentage who breast fed initially		Bases	
Under 20	47	42	280	380
20–24	69	65	739	898
25–29	87	81	598	729
30 or over	86	86	211	337
All first babies*	74	69	1,831	2,347

* Includes some cases where mother's age was not known

2.1.5 Incidence of breast feeding and region

Table 2.6 and Figure 2.6 show that the picture established in the previous surveys of a decline in breast feeding rates as one moves northwards through the country is still apparent in 1985, ranging from 74% in London and the South East to 48% in Scotland. Table 2.6 compares the 1985 figures with those for 1980 and shows that the slight increase overall in the South West and Wales, from 65% to 68%, is more than offset

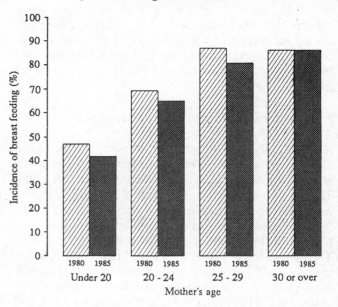

Figure 2.5 Incidence of breast feeding first babies by mother's age (1980 and 1985 Great Britain)

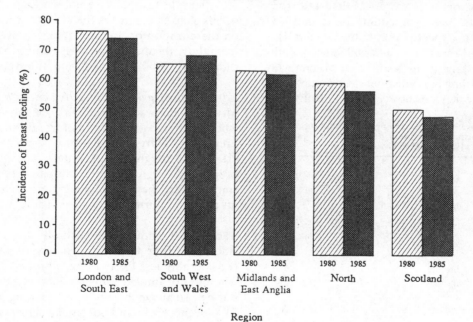

Figure 2.6 Incidence of breast feeding by region (1980 and 1985 Great Britain)

Table 2.6 Incidence of breast feeding by region (1980 and 1985)

Region	First births		Later births		All babies	
	1980	1985	1980	1985	1980	1985
	Percentage who breast fed initially					
London and South East	85	81	69	69	76	74
South West and Wales	75	74	59	63	65	68
Midlands and East Anglia	73	66	56	59	63	62
North	68	63	52	50	59	56
Scotland*	57	53	46	45	50	48
All babies	74	69	58	59	65	64
Bases:						
London and South East	*574*	*747*	*708*	*928*	*1,284*	*1,675*
South West and Wales	*197*	*298*	*286*	*359*	*483*	*657*
Midlands and East Anglia	*345*	*419*	*458*	*541*	*808*	*960*
North	*518*	*628*	*654*	*750*	*1,179*	*1,378*
Scotland*	*722*	*875*	*989*	*1,020*	*1,718*	*1,895*
All babies	*1,831*	*2,347*	*2,377*	*2,875*	*4,224*	*5,223*

* The data for Scotland are weighted to give a national estimate

by small decreases in all the other regions. The overall drop in the incidence of breast feeding among mothers of first babies reflects falling rates in all regions, particularly the Midlands and East Anglia. However, among mothers of later babies the picture was more complex, the rates going up in the South West and Wales and in the Midlands and East Anglia, and down slightly in the North.

2.1.6 Incidence of breast feeding and previous experience of breast feeding

As mentioned earlier, whether or not a mother breast feeds a second or subsequent baby is significantly affected by her experience of feeding her first child. This is shown clearly in Table 2.7. Only 25% of mothers who had not breast fed their first child breast fed their latest baby, compared with 95% of those who had breast fed an earlier child for at least three months. The picture in 1985 is very similar to that in 1980, that is the effect of previous experience does not appear to have changed. This is in contrast to the changes previously noted between 1975 and 1980 when it was found that mothers who had not previously breast fed or had only done so for a short time were less deterred from trying again in 1980 than their counterparts in 1975. Although it cannot be expected that many women who choose to bottle feed their first child will subsequently change to breast feeding, it still seems that women who have tried breast feeding are being deterred from trying again if the first experience is not very successful.

2.1.7 Incidence of breast feeding and mother's working status at about six weeks

At the time of completing the stage 1 questionnaire, when their babies were about six to ten weeks old, mothers were asked whether they were doing any paid work or whether they were on paid or unpaid maternity leave. Only a tiny minority, 5%, were in paid work at this stage, with a further 6% each on paid and unpaid maternity leave. Thus the overwhelming majority (83%) were neither in paid work nor on maternity leave. Although it has been suggested that the increased proportions of women working when their children are very young might affect the proportion of mothers who choose to breast feed, the survey results show no evidence to support this (Table 2.8). Mothers on maternity leave were more likely than other mothers to breast feed; this was the case both among mothers of first babies and of later babies. Overall similar proportions of mothers who were in paid work and who were not working at around six weeks had breast fed initially.

However among mothers of first babies those who were working tended, if anything, to be more likely to breast feed than those who were not working. A later section in this chapter examines the effect of returning to work on the duration of breast feeding. However, it is clear from these results that an early return to work does not significantly inhibit women from breast feeding initially.

2.1.8 Incidence of breast feeding and smoking

Mothers were asked for the first time in the 1985 survey whether they had smoked before, during or after their pregnancy. Thirty-nine per cent of mothers were smokers before pregnancy of whom 24% gave up during pregnancy. High social class was correlated with low smoking rates before pregnancy and high rates of giving up the habit during pregnancy (Table 2.9).

Table 2.10 shows that overall those women who smoked, either before pregnancy or during it, were considerably less likely to have breast fed than women who did not smoke. Only 46% of women who smoked during pregnancy began breast feeding compared with 71% of those who did not smoke. However, smoking is strongly related to social class so it is important to know whether it was the fact that a woman smoked, or merely her social class, which was associated with breast feeding. Comparing the incidence of breast feeding between smokers and non-smokers within each social class group separately, it was still the case that within

Table 2.7 Incidence of breast feeding among mothers of more than one child according to length of time for which first child was breast fed (1980 and 1985 Great Britain)

Length of time for which first child was breast fed	1980	1985	1980	1985
	Percentage who breast fed initially		*Bases:*	
First child bottle fed	28	25	953	1,066
1 week or less	45	45	197	338
More than 1 week, up to 2 weeks	55	59	160	123
More than 2 weeks, up to 4 weeks	68	65	151	167
More than 4 weeks, up to 6 weeks	76	75	154	194
More than 6 weeks, up to 3 months	90	85	230	326
More than 3 months, up to 6 months	91	95	245	271
More than 6 months	96	94	292	415
All second and subsequent babies*	58	59	2,377	2,875

* Includes some cases where details of feeding first child were not known

Table 2.8 Incidence of breast feeding by mother's working status (1980 and 1985 Great Britain)

Mother's working status	First births*	Later births*	All babies		First birth	Later birth	All babies	
	1985	1985	1980	1985	1985	1985	1980	1985
	Percentage who breast fed initially				*Bases:*			
Working	72	57	64	63	103	173	173	276
On maternity leave – paid	80	75	}82	79	219	76	}337	295
unpaid	85	65		80	260	78		338
Not working	66	58	63	61	1,760	2,529	3,699	4,289
All babies†	69	59	65	64	2,347	2,875	4,224	5,223

* 1980 figures not available
† Includes some cases where mother's working status was not known

Table 2.9 Proportion of mothers who smoked before pregnancy, during pregnancy and who gave up during pregnancy (1985 Great Britain)

Social class	Percentage of mothers who smoked:		Base: all mothers	Percentage of mothers who gave up smoking during pregnancy	Base: those who smoked before pregnancy
	before pregnancy	during pregnancy			
I	16	8	307	51	49
II	26	18	1,028	32	268
III Non-manual	28	19	436	35	124
III Manual	41	31	1,666	25	683
IV	41	32	738	23	303
V	53	46	247	13	130
Unclassified	45	38	207	15	93
No partner	64	53	595	17	381
Total	39	30	5,223	24	2,031

Table 2.10 Incidence of breast feeding by smoking and social class (1985 Great Britain)

| Social class | Proportion of women who started breast feeding initially | | | | Bases: | | | |
| | Smoking status before pregnancy: | | Smoking status during pregnancy: | | Smoking status before pregnancy: | | Smoking status during pregnancy: | |
	Non-smoker	Smoker	Non-smoker	Smoker	Non-smoker	Smoker	Non-smoker	Smoker
I	88	81	89	70	258	49	282	24
II	85	69	84	66	760	268	846	182
III Non-manual	82	62	80	59	312	124	355	81
III Manual	66	53	65	50	983	683	1,153	513
IV	62	51	64	45	435	303	504	234
V	49	39	50	35	117	130	134	113
Unclassified	64	44	67	35	114	93	127	79
No partner	45	36	48	32	214	381	280	315
Total	71	52	71	46	3,193	2,031	3,682	1,541

Table 2.11 Perceived financial position when babies were about six weeks old for first and later births (1985 Great Britain)

Perceived financial position	First births	Later births	All babies
	%	%	%
Managing quite well	46	40	43
Just getting by	44	50	47
Getting into difficulties	9	9	9
Other	1	1	1
Base:	2,347	2,875	5,223

every group the smokers had a lower incidence of breast feeding than the non-smokers. Thus smoking during or before pregnancy is associated with a low initial rate of breast feeding.

2.1.9 Incidence of breast feeding and perceived financial position when the babies were about six weeks old
In the 1985 survey mothers were asked how they thought they and their families were managing financially now that they had a new baby. At about six weeks after the birth 43% said they were managing quite well on their money, 47% said they were just getting by and

9% said they were getting into difficulties (Table 2.11). Similar proportions of mothers of first babies and other mothers said they were getting into financial difficulties, but mothers of first babies were more likely to have said they were managing quite well, 46% compared with 40%, and less likely to have said they were just getting by, 44% compared with 50%. This might seem surprising as the biggest financial change to one's circumstances is likely to occur with the first baby, but it may take longer than six to ten weeks for the impact of the change to become apparent.

As one would expect, perceived financial position was strongly related to social class, with those in the highest social classes experiencing fewest financial difficulties (Table 2.12). Within each social class group, mothers of first babies were still more likely than other mothers to be managing quite well.

Because of the close relationship between social class and financial circumstances, it is hardly surprising that the incidence of breast feeding was highest among

Table 2.12 Perceived financial position when babies were about six weeks old by social class (1985 Great Britain)

| Perceived financial position | Social class | | | | | | | | |
	I	II	IIINM	IIIM	IV	V	Unclassified	No partner	Total
	%	%	%	%	%	%	%	%	%
Managing quite well	75	58	46	43	33	24	31	23	43
Just getting by	23	36	47	49	55	62	54	54	47
Getting into difficulties	1	4	6	7	12	14	14	22	9
Other	2	2	1	1	1	–	1	1	1
	100	100	100	100	100	100	100	100	100
Base:	305	1,026	431	1,657	729	244	197	584	5,173

Table 2.13 Incidence of breast feeding by perceived financial position when baby was about 6 weeks old and birth order (1985 Great Britain)

Perceived financial position	First births	Later births	All babies	First births	Later births	All babies
	Percentage who breast fed initially			*Bases:*		
Managing quite well	75	64	69	*1,080*	*1,145*	*2,225*
Just getting by	65	55	60	*1,015*	*1,415*	*2,430*
Getting into difficulties	58	54	56	*200*	*264*	*464*
Other	77	62	71	*32*	*22*	*54*
Total*	69	59	64	*2,347*	*2,875*	*5,223*

* *Includes some cases for whom financial position was not known*

those who felt they were managing quite well financially (69%) and lowest among those who were experiencing difficulties (56%) (Table 2.13). This was true both among mothers of first babies and among mothers of later babies. Controlling for social class revealed that only among mothers in the lowest social classes (IV and V) did financial position have an effect, over and above social class, on whether or not the mother started breast feeding, those with financial difficulties being less likely to have breast fed than the rest.

2.1.10 Estimating separate effects on the incidence of breast feeding

The main socio-demographic variables which have been shown to be associated with the incidence of breast feeding are themselves interrelated. A method of analysis was used on the previous two surveys which takes account of these interrelationships and allows us to make estimates of the incidence of breast feeding for each variable in turn, standardising for the effects of the other interrelated variables. In order to make comparisons with 1980 the same variables have been included in the analysis. However, in 1980 mothers

whose social class could not be classified were excluded from the analysis. In view of the low breast feeding rates among mothers with no partners in 1985 we have included such mothers as a separate group, so we allow for the effect of the other variables on their breast feeding rate. Thus the variables included in the analysis are whether the baby was a first birth or not, social class, the age at which the mother completed her full-time education and region.

Before the standardisation was carried out a better estimate of the incidence of breast feeding was made for each cell of the multi-dimensional table formed by cross-tabulating each of the variables by each other. A model was fitted which takes account of the interrelationships between all the variables and eliminates chance fluctuations due to small numbers in some cells.

The results indicated that each of the four variables included was significantly and independently related to the incidence of breast feeding. Estimates were produced of the incidence of breast feeding for each of the subgroups included and are shown in Table 2.14. From

Table 2.14 Estimated incidence of breast feeding for total sample (1985 Great Britain)

Birth order	Mother's age at finishing full-time education	Region	Social class					
			I	II	IIINM	IIIM	IV & V	Unclassified
			Percentage who breast fed initially					
First births	16 or under	London & SE	84	82	82	71	67	53
		SW & Wales	82	79	78	66	62	47
		Midlands	80	76	76	63	59	44
		North	75	71	70	57	52	37
		Scotland	66	61	60	46	41	28
	17 or 18	London & SE	92	91	91	84	81	71
		SW & Wales	91	89	88	81	78	66
		Midlands	89	87	87	79	75	63
		North	86	84	84	74	70	56
		Scotland	80	77	76	64	60	45
	Over 18	London & SE	96	96	96	92	91	84
		SW & Wales	96	95	94	90	89	81
		Midlands	95	94	94	89	87	79
		North	93	92	92	86	84	74
		Scotland	90	88	88	80	77	64
Later births	16 or under	London & SE	76	72	72	58	54	38
		SW & Wales	72	68	67	53	48	34
		Midlands	69	65	64	50	45	31
		North	63	58	58	43	38	25
		Scotland	52	47	46	32	28	18
	17 or 18	London & SE	87	85	85	75	71	58
		SW & Wales	85	82	81	71	67	52
		Midlands	83	80	79	68	63	49
		North	78	75	74	62	57	42
		Scotland	70	65	65	51	46	32
	Over 18	London & SE	93	93	92	87	85	75
		SW & Wales	92	91	91	84	82	71
		Midlands	91	90	90	83	80	68
		North	89	87	87	78	75	62
		Scotland	84	81	81	70	65	51

this one can see that the highest rate of breast feeding (96%) would be expected among mothers of first babies, who were educated beyond the age of 18, whose partners had professional or managerial occupations and whose babies were born in the South East, as was the case in 1975 and 1980. Conversely the lowest rate (18%) would be expected among mothers having a second or subsequent baby, who left school when they were 16 or less, who had no partner or whose partner's occupation was unclassifiable and whose babies were born in Scotland.

Tables 2.15–2.18 show the standardised and unstandardised rates of breast feeding for each variable in turn. For example the standardised rates of breast feeding for first births and for second and subsequent births are those that would be expected if the two categories were identical in comparison in terms of mother's education, social class and region. In fact the standardised incidence figures for first and later births do not differ from the unstandardised rates, but for the other variables standardisation has reduced the range of results found in the different subgroups. Despite this reduction, the standardised rates are still significantly different for each subgroup. This indicates that although some of the apparent differences between subgroups were due to interrelationships between the variables, all four variables were independently related to the incidence of breast feeding.

2.2 Prevalence of breast feeding

Prevalence of breast feeding refers to the proportion of babies still breast fed at specified ages, even if the babies were also receiving infant formula or solid food. Even if there had been little change in the incidence of breast feeding between 1980 and 1985, mothers could stop breast feeding at different rates, resulting in differences in prevalence of breast feeding among older babies. However, Table 2.19 and Figure 2.7 show this not to be the case. Overall in Great Britain there has

Table 2.15 Estimated incidence of breast feeding by birth order, standardised for social class, mother's education and region, compared with the unstandardised rate (1985 Great Britain)

Birth order	Standardised	Unstandardised
	Percentage who breast fed initially	
First births	69	69
Later births	59	59

Table 2.16 Estimated incidence of breast feeding by social class, standardised for birth order, mother's education and region, compared with the unstandardised rate (1985 Great Britain)

Social class		Standardised	Unstandardised
		Percentage who breast fed initially	
I	Professional	79	87
II	Managerial and technical	75	81
IIINM	Clerical and minor supervisory	75	76
IIIM	Skilled manual	64	61
IV & V	Semi-skilled and unskilled manual	59	54
Unclassified and no partner		46	44

Table 2.17 Estimated incidence of breast feeding by mother's education, standardised for birth order, social class and region, compared with the unstandardised rate (1985 Great Britain)

Mother's age at finishing full-time education	Standardised	Unstandardised
	Percentage who breast fed initially	
16 or under	56	53
17 or 18	72	75
Over 18	85	89

Table 2.18 Estimated incidence of breast feeding by region standardised for birth order, social class and mother's education, compared with the unstandardised rate (1985 Great Britain)

Region	Standardised	Unstandardised
	Percentage who breast fed initially	
London and South East	71	74
South West and Wales	67	68
Midlands and East Anglia	64	62
North	59	56
Scotland	49	48

Figure 2.7 Prevalence of breast feeding in Great Britain: 1980 and 1985

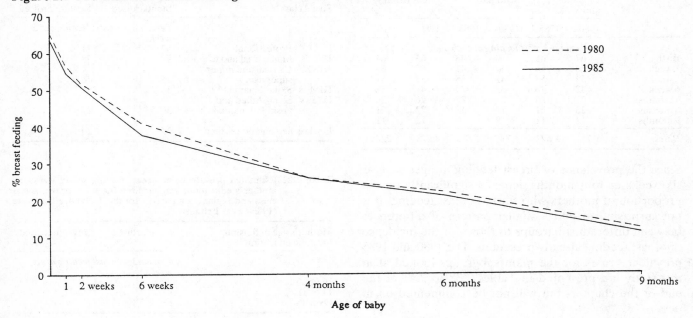

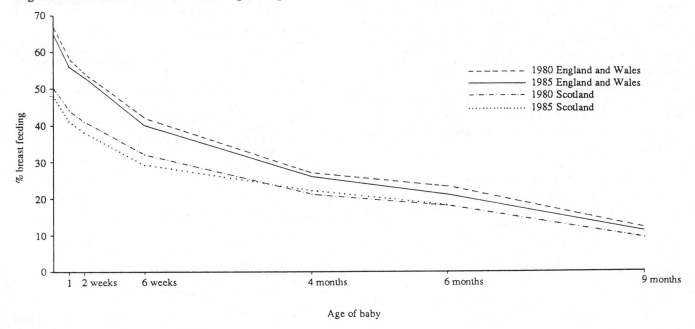

Figure 2.8 Prevalence of breast feeding in England and Wales and in Scotland: 1980 and 1985

Legend:
- – – – – – 1980 England and Wales
- ———— 1985 England and Wales
- –·–·–·– 1980 Scotland
- ············ 1985 Scotland

Y-axis: % breast feeding

X-axis: 1, 2 weeks, 6 weeks, 4 months, 6 months, 9 months

Age of baby

been virtually no change in the prevalence of breast feeding at ages up to nine months. The separate rates for Scotland and England and Wales show a similar picture (Figure 2.8). As in 1980 the rates for Scotland are generally lower than those for England and Wales at all ages, but there has been no significant change over time.

Since 1974 there has been an officially endorsed recommendation that mothers breast feed their babies, preferably for four to six months, but at least for the first few weeks of life. Table 2.19 shows that mothers in Great Britain are nowhere near achieving this aim. Only 51% of mothers breast fed even for as long as two weeks and only 26% breast fed for four months or more.

Table 2.19 Prevalence of breast feeding at ages up to nine months by country (1980 and 1985)

	England and Wales		Scotland		Great Britain	
	1980	1985	1980	1985	1980	1985
	Percentage breast feeding at each age					
Birth	67	65	50	48	65	64
1 week	58	56	44	41	57	55
2 weeks	54	53	41	38	52	51
6 weeks	42	40	32	29	41	38
4 months	27	26	21	22	26	26
6 months	23	21	18	18	22	21
9 months	12	11	9	9	12	11
Bases:	*3,755*	*4,671*	*1,718*	*1,895*	*4,224*	*5,223*

Since the prevalence of breast feeding at ages such as six weeks or four months depends significantly on the proportion of mothers who started breast feeding, it is not surprising to find a similar pattern of differences between different subgroups to those for the incidence of breast feeding already presented. The 1980 and 1985 prevalence rates for the main subgroups looked at in this study are presented in Tables 2.38 to 2.41 at the end of the chapter, but will not be commented on in detail.

A similar analysis to that described in the previous section was carried out to give standardised prevalence rates at six weeks for the same four variables. These results are shown in Tables 2.20 to 2.23.

Table 2.20 Estimated prevalence of breast feeding at six weeks by birth order, standardised for social class, mother's education and region, compared with the unstandardised rate (1985 Great Britain)

Birth order	Standardised	Unstandardised
	Percentage breast feeding at six weeks	
First births	38	39
Later births	38	38

Table 2.21 Estimated prevalence of breast feeding at six weeks by social class, standardised for birth order, mother's education and region, compared with the unstandardised rate (1985 Great Britain)

Social class		Standardised	Unstandardised
		Percentage breast feeding at six weeks	
I	Professional	57	71
II	Managerial and technical	50	58
IIINM	Clerical and minor supervisory	45	46
IIIM	Skilled manual	36	34
IV & V	Semi-skilled and unskilled manual	31	27
Unclassified and no partner		23	20

Table 2.22 Estimated prevalence of breast feeding at six weeks by mother's education, standardised for birth order, social class and region, compared with the unstandardised rate (1985 Great Britain)

Mother's age at finishing full-time education	Standardised	Unstandardised
	Percentage breast feeding at six weeks	
16 or under	29	26
17 or 18	45	48
Over 18	63	73

Table 2.23 Estimated prevalence of breast feeding at six weeks by region, standardised for birth order, social class and mother's education, compared with the unstandardised rate (1985 Great Britain)

Region	Standardised	Unstandardised
	Percentage breast feeding at six weeks	
London and South East	43	47
South West and Wales	46	47
Midlands and East Anglia	37	35
North	33	30
Scotland	30	29

2.3 Duration of breast feeding

In order to separate out the effect of differences in the incidence of breast feeding from differences in the length of time for which mothers who breast feed continue to do so, it is necessary to look separately at those mothers who began breast feeding. The following results therefore relate only to mothers who started breast feeding at all, and show how long they continued breast feeding, even if they were also giving other foods.

Between 1980 and 1985 there has been virtually no change in the length of time for which mothers breast feed. This was the case in Great Britain as a whole and in England and Wales and Scotland separately (Table 2.24 and Figure 2.9). This is in contrast to the increase in the duration of breast feeding observed between 1975 and 1980. In 1985, as in 1980, the duration of breast feeding in Scotland was similar to that in England and Wales and so the overall low levels of the prevalence of breast feeding in Scotland are due to the low initial incidence of breast feeding rather than to those who breast feed doing so for only a short time. In fact, mothers in Scotland were likely to continue breast feeding for longer than those in England and Wales – 45% breast fed for at least four months compared with 40% in England and Wales (Table 2.24).

Table 2.24 Duration of breast feeding for those who were breast fed initially by country (1980 and 1985)

	England and Wales		Scotland		Great Britain	
	1980	1985	1980	1985	1980	1985
	Percentage still breast feeding					
Birth	100	100	100	100	100	100
1 week	88	87	89	85	88	86
2 weeks	81	81	81	79	81	81
6 weeks	63	61	64	60	63	61
4 months	40	40	42	45	40	41
6 months	34	33	36	36	34	33
9 months	18	17	18	20	18	17
Base:	*2,499*	*3,052*	*861*	*918*	*2,734*	*3,319*

Table 2.25 Duration of breast feeding for those who were breast fed initially for first and later births (1980 and 1985 Great Britain)

	First births		Later births		All babies	
	1980	1985	1980	1985	1980	1985
	Percentage still breast feeding					
Birth	100	100	100	100	100	100
1 week	85	83	90	90	88	86
2 weeks	78	76	84	85	81	81
6 weeks	59	56	67	65	63	61
4 months	35	36	45	46	40	41
6 months	29	28	39	38	34	33
9 months	14	14	22	21	18	17
Base:	*1,349*	*1,642*	*1,377*	*1,677*	*2,734*	*3,319*

Tables 2.25–2.28 show figures for the duration of breast feeding by birth order, social class, age at which the mother finished full-time education and region, comparing the 1980 results for Great Britain with those for 1985.

In general the lack of change in the duration of breast feeding compared with 1980 occurred in all the subgroups.

Figure 2.9 Duration of breast feeding for those who were breast fed initially (1980 and 1985 Great Britain)

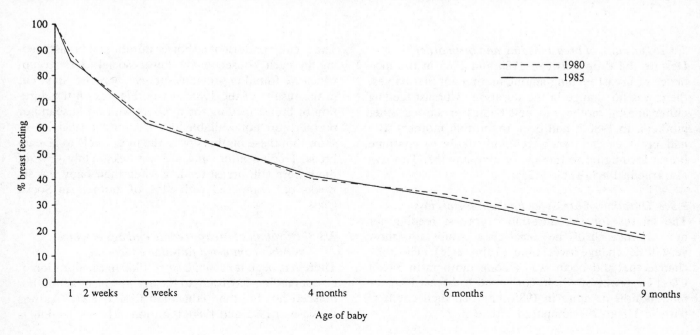

Table 2.26 Duration of breast feeding for those who were breast fed initially by social class (1980 and 1985 Great Britain)

	I		II		IIINM		IIIM		IV and V		IV*	V*	Unclass-ified*	No partner*
	1980	1985	1980	1985	1980	1985	1980	1985	1980	1985	1985	1985	1985	1985
	Percentage still breast feeding													
Birth	100	100	100	100	100	100	100	100	100	100	100	100	100	100
1 week	94	95	91	91	85	88	86	84	83	83	82	85	85	77
2 weeks	91	91	87	86	80	82	79	79	74	75	74	76	79	69
6 weeks	85	81	74	72	62	61	56	56	52	50	51	46	56	43
4 months	67	62	53	54	39	40	32	36	22	27	29	22	39	22
6 months	57	52	46	45	34	33	27	27	15	20	22	17	36	18
9 months	36	27	22	26	18	15	13	14	11	8	9	6	25	11
Base:	293	268	601	830	273	332	1,051	1,009	342	532	425	107	114	235

* 1980 data not available

Table 2.27 Duration of breast feeding for those who were breast fed initially by age at which mother finished full-time education (1980 and 1985 Great Britain)

	Age at which mother finished full-time education							
	16 or under		17 or 18		Over 18		All babies	
	1980	1985	1980	1985	1980	1985	1980	1985
	Percentage still breast feeding							
Birth	100	100	100	100	100	100	100	100
1 week	84	82	90	89	94	95	88	86
2 weeks	76	75	83	83	91	91	81	81
6 weeks	54	50	65	64	84	81	63	61
4 months	29	30	43	40	66	66	40	41
6 months	25	24	34	32	57	56	34	33
9 months	12	12	19	17	32	31	18	17
Base:	1,450	1,633	675	1,013	584	647	2,734	3,319

Table 2.28 Duration of breast feeding for those who were breast fed initially by region (1980 and 1985)

	London and South East		South West and Wales		Midlands and East Anglia		North		Scotland	
	1980	1985	1980	1985	1980	1985	1980	1985	1980	1985
	Percentage still breast feeding									
Birth	100	100	100	100	100	100	100	100	100	100
1 week	88	89	91	88	86	86	87	82	89	85
2 weeks	82	84	84	82	79	80	80	76	81	79
6 weeks	67	64	67	69	56	57	60	54	64	60
4 months	43	43	40	49	37	38	39	32	42	45
6 months	36	36	34	40	33	30	31	26	36	36
9 months	20	18	16	22	17	13	17	16	18	20
Base:	974	1,241	316	449	512	595	696	766	861	918

2.3.1 Duration of breast feeding and birth order

Despite the drop between 1980 and 1985 in the incidence of breast feeding among mothers of first babies, there was no change in the duration of breast feeding either among mothers of first babies or among other mothers. In 1980 it had been found that mothers who had previous children were more likely to continue breast feeding up to the age of nine months. This was also true in 1985 (Table 2.25).

2.3.2 Duration of breast feeding and social class

The figures for the duration of breast feeding for mothers in each of the social class groups also show very little change over time (Table 2.26). The only change that did occur was among mothers in Social Class I – fewer of whom continued to breast feed for nine months or more in 1985 than had their counterparts in 1980: 27% compared with 36%.

The regular pattern of a shorter duration of breast feeding in each consecutively lower social class group, which we found in previous surveys, was also apparent in the results of the 1985 survey. Figures on the duration of breast feeding for mothers with no husband or partner were not available for 1980, but the 1985 figures show that these mothers were the most likely to give up breast feeding after only a few weeks. Only 43% of them were still breast feeding when their baby was six weeks old compared with 81% of mothers in Social Class I.

2.3.3 Duration of breast feeding and age at which mother completed full-time education

There has been no change since 1980 in the duration of breast feeding according to the age at which the mother finished her full-time education (Table 2.27). As was the case in 1975 and 1980, duration of breast feeding is longest among mothers who finished full-time education after the age of 18 and shortest among those who finished at age 16 or below.

2.3.4 Duration of breast feeding and region

Figure 2.10 and Table 2.28 show that in London and the South East and in the Midlands and East Anglia duration of breast feeding did not change between 1980 and 1985. The slight increase in the incidence of breast feeding that occurred in the South West and Wales between 1980 and 1985 was accompanied by an in-crease in the duration of breast feeding for six weeks or longer. This was in contrast to the change observed in the North where the length of time for which mothers continued to breast feed fell. Only 32% of mothers continued to breast feed for as long as four months compared with 39% in 1980 (Table 2.28). In Scotland the duration of breast feeding changed little. However, there was a tendency for Scottish mothers to be less likely than their 1980 counterparts to continue breast feeding for as long as three months, but those that did were more likely to carry on for longer.

Figure 2.10 Duration of breast feeding for those who were breast fed initially for each region (1980 and 1985)

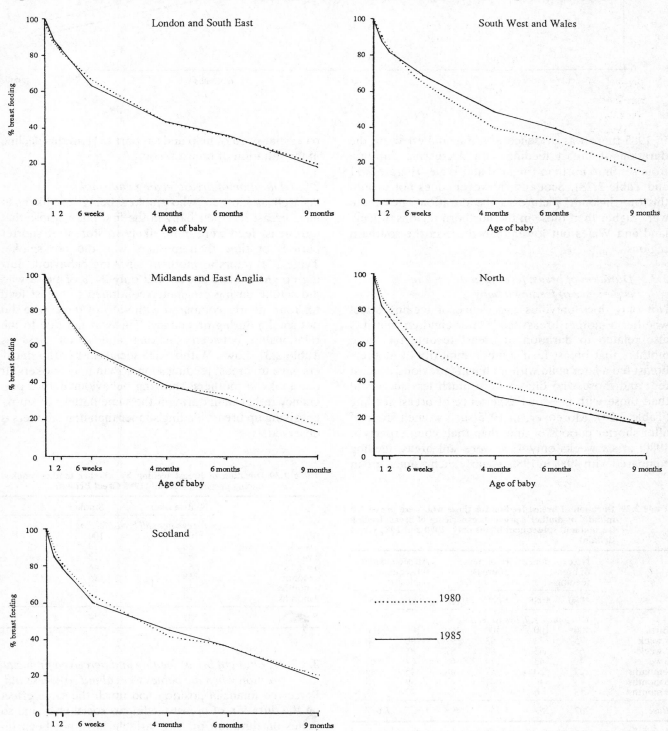

Figure 2.11 Duration of breast feeding for those who were breast fed initially by region (1985)

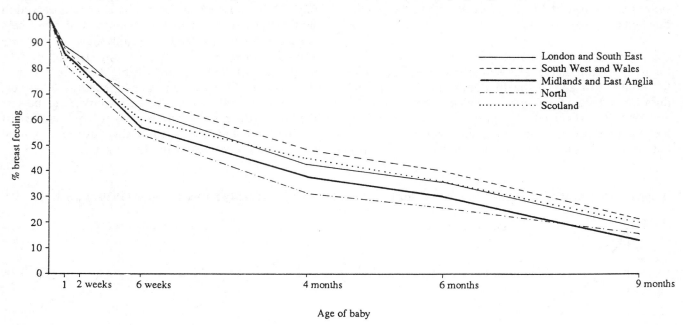

In 1985 there was evidence of a regional effect on the duration of breast feeding with decreasing duration from south to north in England and Wales (Figure 2.11 and Table 2.28). Scotland, however, does not fit into this 'north-south' picture as the duration rates there were higher than those in the northern regions of England and Wales but lower than those in the southern regions.

2.3.5 Duration of breast feeding and previous experience of feeding a baby

Not only does previous experience of feeding affect whether a mother breast feeds later children, but it is also related to duration of breast feeding for those mothers that breast feed. Only a minority of mothers breast fed a later child without having previously breast fed, and those who did so were much less successful than those with previous experience of breast feeding (Table 2.29). Moreover, in 1985 such women stopped after shorter periods of time than their counterparts in 1980: at six weeks only 43% were still breast feeding compared with 49% in 1980. Clearly such women are in

particular need of help and support to stem this decline in the duration of breast feeding.

2.3.6 Duration of breast feeding and smoking

As well as mothers who smoked being less likely to have breast fed their baby in the first place, those that did breast feed were more likely to stop after shorter periods of time than mothers who did not smoke. Table 2.30 refers to mothers' smoking behaviour during pregnancy and shows that only 24% of those who did smoke during pregnancy continued to breast feed for four months compared with 45% of those who did not smoke during pregnancy. This was not due to the relationship between smoking and social class as Table 2.31 shows. Within each social class group smokers gave up breast feeding sooner than non-smokers. If one looks at mothers' smoking behaviour before pregnancy rather than during it the same pattern of smokers giving up breast feeding sooner than non-smokers is observed.

Table 2.30 Duration of breast feeding by whether mother smoked during pregnancy or not (1985 Great Britain)

	Non-smoker	Smoker
	Percentage still breast feeding	
Birth	100	100
1 week	88	79
2 weeks	83	73
6 weeks	65	46
4 months	45	24
6 months	36	19
9 months	19	10
Base:	*2,605*	*714*

2.3.7 Duration of breast feeding and perceived financial position when the babies were about six weeks old

Perceived financial position had much the same effect on the duration of breast feeding as social class and so tables on duration by this variable have not been included.

Table 2.29 Duration of breast feeding for those who were breast fed initially by mother's previous experience of breast feeding (second and subsequent births only, 1980 and 1985 Great Britain)

	No experience of breast feeding		Experience of breast feeding		All second and subsequent babies*	
	1980	1985	1980	1985	1980	1985
	Percentage still breast feeding					
Birth	100	100	100	100	100	100
1 week	75	74	93	92	90	90
2 weeks	65	63	87	87	84	85
6 weeks	49	43	70	68	67	65
4 months	27	20	47	48	45	46
6 months	23	14	41	40	39	38
9 months	13	6	23	22	22	21
Base:	*207*	*157*	*1,169*	*1,498*	*1,377*	*1,677*

* *Includes some cases where it was not known whether the mother had previous experience of breast feeding or not*

Table 2.31 Duration of breast feeding by whether mother smoked during pregnancy or not and social class (1985 Great Britain)

| | Social class | | | | | | | | | | | |
| | I and II | | IIINM | | IIIM | | IV | | V | | Unclassified and no partner | |
	Non-smoker	Smoker	Non-smoker	Smoker	Non-smoker	Smoker	Non-smoker	Smoker	Non-smoker	Smoker	Non-smoker	Smoker
	Percentage still breast feeding											
Birth	100	100	100	100	100	100	100	100	100	100	100	100
1 week	92	88	87	93	86	79	85	74	89	77	86	71
2 weeks	88	81	81	85	81	75	77	66	81	69	79	63
6 weeks	76	66	61	60	60	45	54	40	51	36	55	29
4 months	58	36	40	39	40	23	31	21	26	16	31	10
6 months	49	26	34	23	30	18	23	17	21	8	23	9
9 months	27	15	16	6	15	10	9	11	8	1	16	6
Base:	*961*	*136*	*284*	*48*	*754*	*254*	*321*	*105*	*66*	*40*	*219*	*130*

2.3.8 Duration of breast feeding and mother's working status

Mothers were classified into one of the following five groups according to their working status during the first nine months of their baby's life:

(i) those who were working when the baby was about six weeks old and continued working throughout the rest of the nine months,

(ii) those that did not work at all during the first nine months,

(iii) those that returned to work when the baby was between six weeks and four months old,

(iv) those that returned to work when the baby was between four months and nine months old, and

(v) those whose pattern of work followed some other arrangement.

Overall the duration of breast feeding was similar for all these groups of mothers, regardless of their working status (Table 2.32 and Figure 2.12). There was virtually no difference in the duration of breast feeding be-

tween mothers who did not work at all during the first nine months and those who worked throughout this period. Returning to work did seem to reduce slightly the length of time for which mothers continued to breast feed. For example 34% of mothers who went back to work when their baby was aged between six weeks and four months were still breast feeding when the baby was four months old, compared with 41% of mothers who did not work at all during the first nine months, and 46% of mothers who did not go back to work until after the baby was four months old.

It should be remembered, however, that a mother's working status is related to whether or not she is on maternity leave, which is in turn related to her social class, so it is very difficult to look at the effect of returning to work *per se*. This survey provides no evidence that returning to work significantly shortens the length of time for which a mother breast feeds.

2.3.9 Estimating the separate effects on the duration of breast feeding

The figures for the duration of breast feeding presented in the previous tables are, like those for the incidence

Figure 2.12 Duration of breast feeding for those who were breast fed initially by mother's working status (1985 Great Britain)

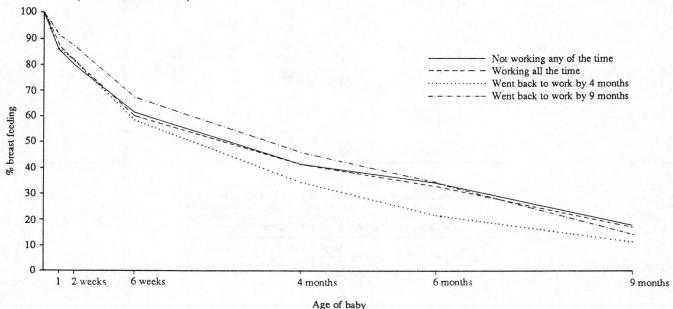

Not working any of the time
Working all the time
Went back to work by 4 months
Went back to work by 9 months

19

and prevalence of breast feeding presented earlier, affected by interrelationships between different variables. A similar maximum likelihood analysis was therefore carried out to estimate the proportion of babies breast fed initially who were still being breast fed at six weeks, controlling for these interrelationships. The results are presented in Tables 2.33 –2.37. Although in 1980 no relationship was found between region and the proportion of babies breast fed at six weeks, preliminary analysis showed that there was evidence of such a relationship in 1985 and so the region variable was included in the analysis. Whereas in the 1980 analysis mothers of second and subsequent births were analysed separately according to whether or not they had any experience of breast feeding this same distinction was not made in the 1985 analysis. This was because once the region variable had been included, to have made the further distinction of whether mothers had any previous experience of breast feeding would have resulted in very few cases in some of the cells in the table produced by cross-tabulating each of the variables with each other.

Table 2.32 Duration of breast feeding by mother's working status during the first nine months (1985 Great Britain)

	Working all the time	Went back to work by four months	Went back to work by nine months	Not working any of the time	Others
	Percentage still breast feeding				
Birth	100	100	100	100	100
1 week	87	88	91	86	90
2 weeks	82	82	87	80	85
6 weeks	60	59	67	61	68
4 months	41	34	46	41	54
6 months	33	22	34	34	44
9 months	17	12	14	18	18
Base:	*121*	*266*	*406*	*2,438*	*90*

Table 2.33 Estimated proportion breast fed at six weeks of those who were breast fed initially (1985 Great Britain)

Birth order	Mother's age at finishing full-time education	Region	Social class					
			I	II	IIINM	IIIM	IV & V	Unclassified
			Percentage still breast feeding at six weeks					
First births	16 or under	London & SE	64	56	48	45	40	36
		SW & Wales	72	64	57	54	48	44
		Midlands	61	52	44	41	36	32
		North	59	50	43	40	35	31
		Scotland	61	32	44	40	36	32
	17 or 18	London & SE	75	67	60	57	52	48
		SW & Wales	81	75	68	66	60	56
		Midlands	72	64	56	54	48	44
		North	70	62	55	52	46	42
		Scotland	71	64	56	53	48	44
	Over 18	London & SE	85	80	75	72	68	64
		SW & Wales	89	85	81	79	75	72
		Midlands	83	78	72	69	64	61
		North	82	77	70	68	63	59
		Scotland	83	78	72	69	64	60
Later births	16 or under	London & SE	73	66	59	56	50	46
		SW & Wales	80	73	67	64	59	55
		Midlands	70	62	55	52	46	42
		North	69	61	53	50	45	41
		Scotland	70	62	55	52	46	42
	17 or 18	London & SE	82	76	70	67	62	58
		SW & Wales	86	82	77	74	70	66
		Midlands	79	73	66	64	58	54
		North	78	72	65	62	57	53
		Scotland	79	73	66	64	58	54
	Over 18	London & SE	90	86	82	80	76	73
		SW & Wales	93	90	87	85	82	80
		Midlands	88	84	80	78	73	70
		North	88	83	78	76	72	69
		Scotland	88	84	79	78	73	70

Table 2.34 Estimated proportion breast fed at six weeks of those who were breast fed initially by birth order, standardised for social class, mother's education and region, compared with the unstandardised rate (1985 Great Britain)

Birth order	Standardised	Unstandardised
	Percentage still breast feeding at six weeks	
First births	55	56
Later births	65	65

Table 2.35 **Estimated proportion breast fed at six weeks of those who were breast fed initially by social class, standardised for birth order, mother's education and region, compared with the unstandardised rate (1985 Great Britain)**

Social class		Standardised	Unstandardised
		Percentage still breast feeding at six weeks	
I	Professional	74	81
II	Managerial and technical	67	72
IIINM	Clerical and minor supervisory	61	61
IIIM	Skilled manual	58	56
IV & V	Semi-skilled and unskilled manual	53	50
Unclassified and no partner		49	47

Table 2.36 **Estimated proportion breast fed at six weeks of those who were breast fed initially by mother's education, standardised for birth order, social class and region, compared with the unstandardised rate (1985 Great Britain)**

Mother's age at finishing full-time education	Standardised	Unstandardised
	Percentage still breast feeding at six weeks	
16 or under	52	50
17 or 18	63	64
Over 18	77	81

Table 2.37 **Estimated proportion breast fed at six weeks of those who were breast fed initially by region, standardised for birth order, social class and mother's education, compared with the unstandardised rate (1985 Great Britain)**

Region	Standardised	Unstandardised
	Percentage still breast feeding at six weeks	
London and South East	61	64
South West and Wales	68	69
Midlands and East Anglia	58	57
North	56	54
Scotland	57	60

Table 2.38 **Prevalence of breast feeding at ages up to nine months for first and later births (1980 and 1985 Great Britain)**

Age of baby	First births		Later births		All babies	
	1980	1985	1980	1985	1980	1985
	Percentage breast feeding at each age					
Birth	74	69	58	60	65	64
1 week	63	57	52	53	57	55
2 weeks	57	53	49	50	52	51
6 weeks	43	39	39	38	41	38
4 months	26	25	26	27	26	26
6 months	21	19	23	22	22	21
9 months	10	10	13	12	12	11
Base:	*1,831*	*2,347*	*2,377*	*2,875*	*4,224*	*5,223*

Table 2.39 **Prevalence of breast feeding at ages up to nine months by social class (1980 and 1985 Great Britain)**

Age of baby	I		II		IIINM		IIIM		IV and V		IV*	V*	Unclassified*	No partner
	1980	1985	1980	1985	1980	1985	1980	1985	1980	1985	1985	1985	1985	1985
	Percentage breast feeding at each age													
Birth	87	87	78	81	77	76	59	61	52	54	58	43	55	39
1 week	82	83	71	73	65	67	51	51	43	44	47	36	46	30
2 weeks	80	79	68	69	62	62	47	48	38	40	43	33	43	27
6 weeks	74	71	58	58	48	46	33	34	27	27	29	20	30	16
4 months	59	54	41	43	30	30	19	21	11	14	16	9	20	8
6 months	50	45	36	37	26	24	16	16	8	11	12	7	19	6
9 months	31	23	17	21	14	11	8	8	6	4	5	2	13	4
Base:	*335*	*307*	*769*	*1,028*	*335*	*436*	*1,769*	*1,666*	*659*	*985*	*738*	*247*	*207*	*595*

* 1980 data not available

Table 2.40 Prevalence of breast feeding by age at which mother finished full-time education (1980 and 1985 Great Britain)

Age of baby	Age at which mother finished full-time education							
	16 or under		17 or 18		Over 18		All babies	
	1980	1985	1980	1985	1980	1985	1980	1985
	Percentage breast feeding at each age							
Birth	55	53	76	75	89	89	65	64
1 week	46	43	68	66	84	85	57	55
2 weeks	42	39	63	63	81	82	52	51
6 weeks	30	26	49	48	75	73	41	38
4 months	16	15	33	30	59	59	26	26
6 months	14	12	26	24	51	50	22	21
9 months	7	6	14	13	28	28	12	11
Base:	2,632	3,110	892	1,346	657	725	4,224	5,223

Table 2.41 Prevalence of breast feeding by region (1980 and 1985 Great Britain)

Age of baby	London and South East		South West and Wales		Midlands and East Anglia		North		Scotland	
	1980	1985	1980	1985	1980	1985	1980	1985	1980	1985
	Percentage breast feeding at each age									
Birth	76	74	65	68	63	62	59	56	50	48
1 week	67	67	60	60	54	53	51	46	45	41
2 weeks	62	63	55	56	50	49	47	42	41	38
6 weeks	51	47	44	47	35	35	35	30	32	29
4 months	33	32	26	34	23	23	23	18	21	22
6 months	27	26	22	27	21	11	18	14	18	17
9 months	15	13	10	15	11	8	10	9	9	9
Base:	1,284	1,675	483	657	808	960	1,179	1,378	1,718	1,895

3 Influences on choice of method of feeding

3.1 Introduction

The previous surveys have shown that the most important decisions about whether to breast feed are taken for the first child. Only a minority of women who choose bottle feeding change to breast feeding for their later children. Those who breast feed their first child successfully generally continue to do so for all their children and it is only those who breast feed their first child for a short time who may change to bottle feeding subsequently. The previous surveys have therefore paid particular attention to the choices made by mothers of first babies.

The 1975 survey examined in some detail the influences on their choice, from which it was concluded that social and cultural factors were extremely important. Many of the attitudes that affected women's choices were likely to have been formed in childhood or adolescence, long before the first pregnancy. Although some mothers would have decided on a method of feeding even before they became pregnant or almost as soon as they knew they were pregnant, many would not have made a definite decision before they first came into contact with the health professionals responsible for their care during pregnancy. The health professionals can therefore reasonably be expected to establish early in pregnancy whether the pregnant woman has already made a firm decision, and if not to discuss methods of feeding so that she can make an informed choice.

In this chapter we therefore look particularly at mothers' accounts of their contacts with the health professionals and voluntary organisations providing care and advice for women during pregnancy.

3.2 Choice of method of feeding

In 1985 all except 6% of women said that they had decided before the birth on their method of feeding; 61% planned to breast feed and 33% to bottle feed –

similar proportions to the 1980 figures. Among mothers of first babies 67% planned to breast feed, 25% planned to bottle feed and 7% were undecided before the birth. Table 3.1 shows the powerful effect of previous experience on the intentions of mothers of second and subsequent babies. However, there is some evidence that mothers in 1985 were more likely to be deterred by previous unsuccessful attempts at breast feeding than their counterparts were in 1980 – a reverse of the trend between 1975 and 1980. Even among mothers who had breast fed for six weeks or more, slightly fewer planned to breast feed again in 1985 than in 1980, although the vast majority of these women did plan to breast feed again.

As in 1980, most mothers (95%) who had decided on their method of feeding before the birth carried out their intentions (Table 3.2). Those who appeared to have changed their mind from breast feeding to bottle feeding were more likely to have reported having had problems with the birth.

Tables 3.3 and 3.4 show the reasons for choosing to breast feed and bottle feed respectively. The 1980 figures are shown for comparison and are very similar. It should be noted that in 1985 the mothers who choose to breast feed mentioned fewer reasons for their choice and so all the 1985 proportions are somewhat lower. Also, since mothers were asked to write in their reasons, rather than to choose responses from a list, the answers were coded in the office and differences in coding between 1980 and 1985 may cause some fluctuation in the figures.

Nevertheless, the overall pattern of reasons is clear: by far the most frequently mentioned reason for choosing to breast feed was that breast feeding is thought to be best for the baby. The next most common reason was that breast feeding is more convenient. The most com-

Table 3.1 Mother's intended method of feeding according to previous experience of breast feeding and birth order (1980 and 1985 Great Britain)

Intended method of feeding	First birth		Later birth								All babies	
			No experience of breast feeding		Breast fed for:				All later births			
					Less than 6 weeks		6 weeks or more					
	1980	1985	1980	1985	1980	1985	1980	1985	1980	1985	1980	1985
	%	%	%	%	%	%	%	%	%	%	%	%
Breast	70	67	22	20	53	45	91	87	55	55	61	61
Bottle	22	25	71	74	40	46	6	10	39	40	32	33
Had not decided	8	7	7	6	7	9	3	3	6	5	7	6
	100	100	100	100	100	100	100	100	100	100	100	100
Base:	*1,831*	*2,347*	*879*	*924*	*679*	*704*	*835*	*1,248*	*2,377*	*2,875*	*4,224*	*5,223*

Table 3.2 Proportion of mothers who actually fed their babies in the way they had planned (1980 and 1985 Great Britain)

Planned method	1980	1985	1980	1985
			Bases:	
Breast	97	96	*2,592*	*3,156*
Bottle	94	94	*1,348*	*1,726*
All who had decided on method before birth	96	95	*3,940*	*4,882*

Table 3.3 Mother's reasons for planning to breast feed according to birth order (1980 and 1985 Great Britain)

Mother's reasons	First births		Later births		All babies	
	1980	1985	1980	1985	1980	1985
	%	%	%	%	%	%
Breast feeding is best for the baby	87	86	74	70	80	78
Breast feeding is more convenient	38	30	41	36	40	33
Breast feeding is natural	26	19	19	15	23	17
Breast feeding is cheaper	22	15	23	16	22	16
Closer bond between mother and baby	24	22	21	20	22	21
Mother's own experience	..	..	29	30	15	15
Breast feeding is best for mother	9	6	8	6	8	6
Cannot overfeed by breast	3	0	2	0	2	0
Influenced by medical personnel	2	3	1	1	2	2
Influenced by friends or relatives	2	2	1	1	2	2
No particular reason	1	2	2	1	2	2
Other reasons	1	1	2	4	2	3
*Base:**	*1,281*	*1,516*	*1,303*	*1,509*	*2,593*	*3,025*

* Percentages do not add up to 100 as some mothers gave more than one reason

Table 3.4 Mother's reasons for planning to bottle feed according to birth order (1980 and 1985 Great Britain)

Mother's reasons	First births		Later births		All babies	
	1980	1985	1980	1985	1980	1985
	%	%	%	%	%	%
Other people can feed baby with bottle	44	45	35	35	38	38
Mother's own previous experience	..	..	47	47	34	31
Did not like the idea of breast feeding	28	33	21	18	23	23
Would be embarrassed to breast feed	17	10	9	4	11	6
You can see how much the baby has had	16	8	8	6	10	6
Medical reasons for not breast feeding	3	4	4	4	4	4
Expecting to return to work soon	5	7	2	2	3	4
Persuaded by other people	3	2	2	1	2	1
No particular reason	11	7	4	3	6	4
Other reasons	6	10	4	5	5	6
*Base:**	*403*	*525*	*940*	*1,047*	*1,348*	*1,572*

* Percentages do not add up to 100 as some mothers gave more than one reason

mon reason given for choosing bottle feeding was that other people could feed the baby, although mothers of second and subsequent babies most frequently cited their previous experience. Mothers of first babies who chose to bottle feed were particularly likely to say that they did not like the idea of breast feeding.

3.3 Contact with health professionals during the antenatal period

3.3.1 Antenatal checkups
Almost all mothers (99%) reported receiving antenatal care during their pregnancy. Most were likely to have encountered several different health professionals during pregnancy and many received antenatal care at more than one place, since shared-care schemes are now widespread. In general women first contact their general practitioner who makes arrangements for their antenatal care. Thereafter, there is likely to be contact with at least one midwife and with an obstetrician. Many women will see several midwives, pupil midwives, consultants and junior doctors during the course of their pregnancy, in addition to their GP. Because of this it is not realistic to expect women to remember who they saw and what was said by everyone. The questionnaire therefore asked a number of rather general questions that were thought on the basis of the previous surveys to be particularly important.

Women were asked whether during visits for antenatal checkups they had been asked how they intended to feed the baby. Although 88% said they had been asked it is still noteworthy that 12% said that they had not been asked and that this proportion was not significantly lower among women having a first baby (10%). However, this is a slight improvement on the 1980 figure of 16% of mothers who said they had not been asked how they intended to feed the baby.

Since being asked about plans could mean no more than ticking a box on a form at the booking visit, this question was followed by asking mothers whether during their antenatal visits there had been any discussion about feeding. Table 3.5 shows that overall only 41% of mothers had both been asked about their plans and had a discussion about feeding – not significantly different from the 1980 figure of 39%. However, the figure was higher among women having their first baby (49%) and compares somewhat more favourably with the 1980 figure of 45%.

As on the previous two surveys we examined whether women said during pregnancy they had planned to breast feed in relation to whether they had been asked about their plans or had discussions about feeding during antenatal visits. Table 3.6 shows a very similar picture to 1980: the lowest proportion planning to breast feed was among those who had not been asked their plans or had had no discussion about feeding. Among those who had been asked there was no difference by whether or not there had been a discussion about feeding.

These results might be taken to mean that discussions about methods of feeding have no effect on women's choice of method, but it can be argued that such discussions have two broad aims. First, to ensure, particularly for those in their first pregnancy, that women have sufficient information about both breast and bottle feeding to make an informed choice. Without some discussion the health professionals cannot distinguish between those women who have definitely decided on their method and those who are still unsure. Second, women need information about their chosen method in order to feed their baby successfully by whichever method they have chosen. However, no further questions were asked about the discussions and so we do not know what the content of such discussions was.

3.3.2 Antenatal classes

It may of course be argued that discussions about feeding should take place at antenatal classes rather than during visits for checkups. But this ignores the fact that not all women attend such classes, particularly if they are expecting a second or subsequent child. Yet, as we have seen, some of these women will be breast feeding for the first time or have had problems breast feeding an earlier child and so be in particular need of help and advice. Altogether only 44% of mothers said they had attended antenatal class, but the proportion among mothers of first babies was 71% compared with 22% of those having a later baby. These proportions are slightly higher than the corresponding figures for 1980 of 67% and 18% respectively. Yet despite some increase in attendance at antenatal classes fewer women having first babies are choosing to breast feed and there was no change among those having a later baby.

Table 3.5 Whether mothers were asked about their plans or had discussions about feeding during visits for antenatal check-ups according to birth order (1980 and 1985 Great Britain)

	First births		Later births		All babies	
	1980	1985	1980	1985	1980	1985
	%	%	%	%	%	%
Not asked about plans, no discussion	12	10	17	11	15	11
Asked about plans, no discussion	42	41	47	53	45	47
Not asked about plans, had discussion	1	0	1	1	1	1
Asked about plans, had discussion	45	49	35	35	39	41
	100	100	100	100	100	100
Base:	1,823	2,347	2,368	2,875	4,206	5,223

Table 3.6 Proportion of mothers who planned to breast feed by whether they had been asked their plans or discussed feeding the baby according to birth order (1980 and 1985 Great Britain)

	First births		Later births		All babies	
	1980	1985	1980	1985	1980	1985
	Percentage planning to breast feed					
Not asked about plans, no discussion	60	60	44	45	50	52
Asked about plans, no discussion	71	70	57	57	63	62
Had discussion*	71	67	57	55	64	62
Total	70	67	55	55	61	60
Bases:						
Not asked about plans, no discussion	223	239	395	314	618	553
Asked about plans, no discussion	754	929	1,093	1,484	1,847	2,413
*Had discussion**	855	1,128	887	1,010	1,757	2,138
Total	1,831	2,347	2,377	2,875	4,224	5,223

* Numbers too small to show those who were not asked their plans separately

Since relatively few mothers of second and subsequent babies had attended antenatal classes it was decided to restrict further analysis to mothers of first babies.

As was the case in 1980, attendance at antenatal classes by women expecting their first baby was strongly associated with social class, attendance rates generally falling across the social class groups (Table 3.7).

Table 3.7 Proportion of mothers of first babies who attended antenatal classes by social class (1980 and 1985 Great Britain)

Social class	First births		Bases:	
	1980	1985	*1980*	*1985*
	Percentage attending antenatal classes			
I	90	92	*138*	*136*
II	84	84	*311*	*444*
IIINM	83	86	*179*	*213*
IIIM	65	74	*742*	*703*
IV	}56	63}63	}266	*283*
V		64		*103*
Unclassified	}33	59}48	}195	*81*
No partner		43		*383*
All first births	67	71	*1,831*	*2,347*

Most mothers of first babies said they had attended antenatal classes held at a local clinic or GP's surgery (60%) or a hospital (43%), but a (4%) minority attended classes run by another organisation such as the National Childbirth Trust.

However, not all antenatal classes cover infant feeding; some deal exclusively with relaxation and preparation for the birth. But in 1985, as in 1980, 86% of mothers of first babies who had attended antenatal classes said that talks or discussions about infant feeding had been included. In addition such mothers were asked whether they had been told about the advantages of breast feed-

Table 3.8 Proportions of mothers of first babies who attended antenatal classes receiving certain types of advice (1980 and 1985 Great Britain)

	1980	1985
	Percentage receiving advice	
Received talks or discussions about feeding babies	87	86
Were told about the advantages of breast feeding	84	83
Were taught how to make up a bottle	63	59
Base: Mothers of first babies who attended antenatal classes	*1,228*	*1,657*

ing and whether they had been taught how to make up a bottle. Table 3.8 shows that a similar proportion of mothers had been told about the advantages of breast feeding in 1985 as in 1980, but slightly fewer had been taught how to make up a bottle: 59% compared with 63% in 1980. More mothers of first babies, however, chose to bottle feed in 1985 than in 1980.

As in 1980 attendance at antenatal classes was associated with a higher than average likelihood of planning to breast feed among women having a first baby: 76% of those who attended classes said they planned to breast feed compared with 47% of those who did not attend classes. Since the intention to breast feed and attendance at antenatal classes are both strongly associated with social class, we examined the relationship between feeding intentions and attendance at classes for each social class separately (Table 3.9). This shows that within each social class mothers who attended antenatal classes were more likely to plan to breast feed than those who did not, and the difference between the two groups was more marked among the lower than the higher social class mothers.

However, these results do not show whether antenatal classes have influenced some mothers to breast feed who might otherwise not have done so, since we do not know what their plans were before attendance at the classes. It is equally plausible to suppose that women who were already planning to breast feed were more likely than others to attend classes. Nevertheless, it remains the case that women in the lowest social classes or without a partner are both least likely to breast feed and to attend antenatal classes. Possibly more effort should be made during visits for antenatal checkups to ensure such women have adequate help and advice about feeding.

3.3.3 Home visits during the antenatal period

Although it is official policy for all expectant mothers to be visited at home by a midwife before the birth, when resources are stretched such visits may occur only if a woman is planning to have a home delivery or to stay in hospital for only a short period after the birth of her baby. A few antenatal visits are made to mothers who are ill or otherwise unable to attend for antenatal check-ups. In the case of women planning a home delivery or early discharge, home visits by a midwife enable the woman to get to know the midwife who will be

Table 3.9 Proportion of mothers of first babies intending to breast feed by social class and whether attended antenatal classes (1985 Great Britain)

Social class	Attended classes	Did not attend classes	Total	Attended classes	Did not attend classes	Total
	Percentage intending to breast feed			*Bases:*		
I	90	85	90	*125*	*10*	*136*
II	88	75	86	*375*	*69*	*444*
IIINM	85	74	84	*184*	*29*	*213*
IIIM	72	51	67	*517*	*185*	*702*
IV	71	55	65	*178*	*105*	*283*
V	61	36	52	*65*	*37*	*103*
Unclassified	66	42	56	*47*	*33*	*80*
No partner	51	29	38	*163*	*218*	*382*
All first births	76	47	67	*1,655*	*687*	*2,343*

Table 3.10 Proportion of mothers receiving antenatal home visits by midwives and health visitors according to birth order (1980 and 1985 Great Britain)

Visit made by:	First births		Later births		All babies	
	1980	1985	1980	1985	1980	1985
	Proportion receiving antenatal home visits					
Midwife	35	44	50	51	43	48
Health visitor	19	15	22	17	21	16
Either	44	52	59	59	53	56
Base:	*1,831*	*2,377*	*2,347*	*2,875*	*4,224*	*5,223*

visiting daily after the birth until the baby is ten days old. In some areas home visits are made by health visitors in order to establish contact with the expectant mothers and help to build up a relationship. This may be important after the birth of the baby in that the mother will already have someone she knows to whom she can turn for help and advice.

As was the case in 1980, all mothers who took part in the 1985 survey were asked whether a midwife or health visitor had visited them at home in connection with their pregnancy. Overall, 56% of mothers had received an antenatal visit, a slight increase on the 53% who had received such a visit in 1980 (Table 3.10). Mothers expecting their first baby were more likely to have been visited by a midwife than previously, but there was no change in the likelihood of such a visit for other mothers. All mothers were, however, less likely to have been visited by a health visitor before the birth in 1985 than in 1980.

Since the most common reason for home visits during pregnancy is in connection with home deliveries and early discharges, the proportion of women receiving home visits is likely to be influenced by their plans for delivery and length of hospital stay. As home deliveries in 1985 were a very small proportion of all deliveries, less than 1%, we have looked only at the relationship between home visits and the length of time the mother stayed in hospital. For mothers having their first baby it was more common in 1985 than in 1980 to be booked for discharge after 48 hours and more of them received a home visit by a midwife. As in 1980, all mothers, irrespective of whether they were expecting a first baby or not, were more likely to have received an antenatal home visit if they had stayed in hospital for two days or less than if they had stayed in for longer: 63% of the former received a home visit compared with 53% of the latter.

Although there is no particular reason to expect an association between receiving a home visit and planning to breast feed, such a relationship was found in 1985, but not in 1980. Among mothers expecting their first baby 70% of those who had a visit were planning to breast feed, significantly more than the 65% of mothers who had not had a visit. The corresponding figures among mothers expecting their second or subsequent baby were 58% and 51% respectively.

3.4 Literature containing information on feeding babies
As well as having personal contact with health professionals during their pregnancy, another source of information and advice on feeding methods for expectant mothers is books and pamphlets. Such literature may have some influence on mothers' choice of feeding method. For the first time in the 1985 survey all mothers were asked whether they had been given a copy of *The Pregnancy Book*, a free publication on pregnancy and child care, which includes information and advice on how to feed babies. In England and Wales this book is produced by the Health Education Council. In Scotland the equivalent book is called *The Book of the Child*, produced by the Scottish Health Education Group. Six per cent of mothers could not remember what they had been given in the way of books or pamphlets, but of those who could, 86% remembered receiving a copy of one of the above books. The proportion saying they had received a copy was higher among mothers expecting their first baby than among other mothers: 90% compared with 83%. Whether or not mothers received the book did not vary significantly according to their social background.

We examined whether mothers said they intended to breast feed according to whether they had been given a copy of the book or not. Among mothers expecting their first baby, those who had received the book were more likely to be planning to breast feed than those who had not, 69% compared with 60%. There was no such difference among mothers expecting second or subsequent babies. This does not necessarily imply that reading the book persuaded mothers expecting their first baby to breast feed – they may well have already made up their mind to do so before they read the book. The book does, however, contain useful advice on whichever method of feeding the mother decides upon.

In addition mothers were asked whether they had been given any other free books or pamphlets which included information about feeding babies. The majority had: 88% of those expecting their first baby and 75% of those expecting a later baby. Again there was an association between reporting receiving such pamphlets and planning to breast feed, but only among mothers expecting their first baby. Only a very small proportion of mothers said they had not been given any free literature at all about feeding babies; 2% of those expecting their first baby and 7% of the rest.

3.5 Lessons on parentcraft at school
Nowadays many schools include lessons on parentcraft and child development as part of the curriculum. Such lessons are another source of information to future mothers which may affect whether they decide to breast feed or not. In the 1985 survey all mothers who took

part were asked whether they had had any lessons on parentcraft or child development or anything similar when they were at school. No further questions were asked about the content of such lessons so we do not know what was covered or in how much detail. Whether or not women had had such lessons was strongly related to their social class and the age at which they finished their full-time education. Women in lower social classes who left school at the minimum age were most likely to have attended such classes, probably because such lessons are often only offered to less academic pupils. After having controlled for social background characteristics, having these lessons at school was not associated with intentions to breast feed.

4 Influences on the duration of breast feeding

4.1 Introduction

The previous chapter showed that for mothers who started breast feeding, there was little difference in the length of time for which they continued in 1985 compared with 1980. Thus 19% of mothers who started breast feeding had stopped within two weeks, and 39% had stopped within six weeks. The previous surveys showed that mothers who gave up breast feeding in the early weeks did not generally do so from choice; most had encountered problems and had given up reluctantly. The previous surveys had shown clearly that events around the time of the birth and soon after were strongly associated with success or failure of breast feeding in the early weeks. In particular certain hospital practices could affect the outcome of breast feeding. This chapter examines mothers' reasons for stopping breast feeding and the extent to which the factors shown to be important on the previous surveys are still affecting the success of breast feeding, particularly in the early weeks.

4.2 Reasons for stopping breast feeding

All mothers who had breast fed at all were asked to give reasons for stopping when they did. Table 4.1 shows that their reasons varied according to the length of time for which they had breast fed, as they did in 1980. The most frequently given reason at any age was insufficient milk. We know from the previous surveys that this did not necessarily mean that mothers were unable to produce sufficient milk. Faced with a baby who appeared to be crying from hunger, mothers would assume they did not have enough milk, and even if this was the case, they often did not know what might be done to increase their milk supply and thus abandoned breast feeding.

Other problems featured prominently among the reasons given for stopping breast feeding in the first week or so such as sore nipples or the baby not sucking properly. Mothers with these kinds of problems, or inverted nipples or engorgement, are likely either to overcome them or to give up breast feeding, and so such problems do not feature as reasons for stopping breast feeding beyond the early weeks. The length of time breast feeding took became a more common reason at later stages. However, only among mothers who had breast fed for longer than four months was breast feeding for as long as intended the dominant reason.

Table 4.1 Reasons given by mothers for stopping breast feeding at different ages (1980 and 1985 Great Britain)

Reason for stopping breast feeding	Baby's age when breast feeding ceased: Less than 1 week		1 week but less than 2 weeks		2 weeks but less than 6 weeks		6 weeks but less than 2 months		2 months but less than 3 months		3 months but less than 4 months		4 months but less than 9 months	
	1980	1985	1980	1985	1980	1985	1980	1985	1980	1985	1980	1985	1980	1985
	Percentage giving reason													
Insufficient milk	36	29	58	50	68	63	68	74	74	64	65	60	32	31
Painful breasts or nipples	24	26	25	28	15	17	12	10	10	11	8	8	1	4
Baby would not suck/ rejected breast	30	24	14	16	8	6	5	5	4	9	9	9	17	26
Breast feeding took too long/tiring	7	6	12	7	17	16	14	17	14	15	20	11	8	8
Mother was ill	5	10	6	15	5	7	7	9	8	7	9	6	6	5
Did not like breast feeding	9	12	2	4	2	4	1	3	–	1	–	3	1	0
Domestic reasons	3	4	3	8	4	9	5	6	5	7	9	9	5	4
Mother had inverted nipples	7	4	3	2	1	1	1	–	–	0	–	1	–	–
Baby was ill	2	6	5	4	2	6	3	1	5	6	3	3	1	1
Baby could not be fed by others	1	1	3	2	2	2	2	4	2	3	3	2	7	7
Embarrassment	1	1	2	1	1	2	–	2	1	3	3	1	1	0
Returning to work	1	–	–	1	1	2	1	2	6	6	2	6	6	10
Had breast fed long enough/as long as intended	–	0	1	0	–	0	5	–	4	2	6	11	37	45
Other reasons	4	6	4	4	3	4	6	4	5	12	13	9	26	6
Base: all breast fed babies	*336*	*444*	*182*	*190*	*491*	*652*	*171**	*224**	*215**	*260**	*182**	*183**	*552**	*763**

* Bases are the reweighted numbers
Percentages do not add up to 100 as most mothers gave more than one reason

Table 4.2 Length of time breast feeding mothers stayed in hospital by birth order (1980 and 1985 Great Britain)

Length of stay	First births		Later births		All babies	
	1980	1985	1980	1985	1980	1985
	%	%	%	%	%	%
2 days or less	4	7	41	53	22	30
3–5 days	22	44	29	29	26	36
6 or 7 days	41	32	17	10	29	21
8–10 days	28	14	10	6	19	10
More than 10 days	5	3	3	2	4	2
	100	100	100	100	100	100
*Base:**	*1,346*	*1,627*	*1,349*	*1,654*	*2,703*	*3,281*

* Does not include home births

These results show that, as in 1980, many women were stopping breast feeding earlier than they would have liked because of a variety of problems, most of which appear to be preventable or at least surmountable. It is sometimes suggested that mothers are citing problems as acceptable excuses for giving up breast feeding, but the survey gives little support to this view. It was clear from comments on the questionnaires that many mothers were very upset about stopping breast feeding and took this as a personal failure which reflected on their adequacy as a mother.

4.3 Breast feeding in hospital
In 1985 almost all babies were delivered in hospital. Thus for most women breast feeding starts off in hospital. Events occurring during labour and delivery and the period immediately after the birth affect whether breast feeding gets off to a good start and the previous surveys have examined this period in some detail. Table 4.2 shows that in 1985 mothers were staying in hospital for somewhat shorter periods of time than in 1980, which gives hospital staff less time to ensure that mothers are confident about breast feeding and to help with problems that frequently occur in the early days, particularly for those breast feeding for the first time.

One indication of how successful hospitals are in establishing breast feeding is whether mothers who started breast feeding are still doing so on discharge from hospital. Table 4.3 shows that as in 1980 15% of women who started breast feeding had given up before they left hospital. Since altogether 19% gave up in the first two weeks, only 4% gave up in the remainder of the first two weeks following discharge. These results do not support the view that women manage to breast feed while in hospital only to stop when they get home and

less help is available. The steepest drop in the prevalence of breast feeding is in the first week of life, so the period in hospital is particularly important.

4.4 Events during labour and delivery
The two previous surveys showed that events occurring during labour and delivery can affect the initiation of breast feeding. Faced with complications affecting either her or her baby a mother who had initially planned to breast feed may change her mind. In fact almost all the women who did not carry out their intention to breast feed had had some problems around the time of the birth, such as caesarian delivery or a low birth-weight baby. Nevertheless, many mothers experiencing these sorts of problems did start breast feeding, but as we found previously, they were more likely than other mothers to stop breast feeding in the first few weeks. Because very few mothers who had planned to breast feed did not in fact do so initially, the next few sections will look at factors which are associated with giving up breast feeding in the first two weeks.

Although we asked questions about all types of analgesia received during labour, little effect of these on breast feeding was found on the previous surveys. However, having a general anaesthetic was associated with stopping breast feeding in the first two weeks. Similarly the type of delivery most associated with problems with breast feeding was a caesarian section. In 1985, 7% of women reported having had a general anaesthetic and 11% a caesarian delivery. However, in 1985 it had become somewhat more common to have a caesarian under epidural rather than a general anaesthetic and so we could examine whether the anaesthetic or the type of delivery had most effect on breast feeding.

Table 4.3 Proportion of mothers who stopped breast feeding before leaving hospital by birth order (1980 and 1985 Great Britain)

Method of feeding on discharge from hospital	First births		Later births		All babies	
	1980	1985	1980	1985	1980	1985
	%	%	%	%	%	%
Breast feeding:	81	81	88	89	85	85
Breast feeding completely	72	70	76	77	74	73
Breast and bottle feeding	9	11	12	12	11	12
Stopped breast feeding in hospital	19	19	12	11	15	15
	100	100	100	100	100	100
*Base:**	*1,346*	*1,627*	*1,349*	*1,654*	*2,703*	*3,281*

* Does not include home births

Table 4.4 Proportion of mothers who had stopped breast feeding within two weeks by whether they had a general anaesthetic and/or caesarian delivery (1985 Great Britain)

Type of delivery	Had general anaesthetic	Had other or no anaesthetic	All babies	Had general anaesthetic	Had other or no anaesthetic	All babies
	Percentage stopping breast feeding within two weeks			*Bases:*		
Caesarian	27	20	25	*215*	*106*	*321*
Other delivery	(1)	19	19	*15*	*2,872*	*2,887*
All babies	27	19	19	*230*	*2,978*	*3,319**

* Includes some cases where type of delivery or anaesthesia was not known

Altogether 25% of women who had had a caesarian delivery stopped breast feeding within two weeks, as did 27% of those who had had a general anaesthetic. Table 4.4 compares the proportion of mothers who stopped breast feeding in the first two weeks by the type of delivery they had and whether or not they had a general anaesthetic. Women who had a caesarian delivery either had a general anaesthetic or an epidural. Table 4.4 reveals that of those having a caesarian delivery, those who had it under an epidural were less likely than those who had it under a general anaesthetic to stop breast feeding within two weeks; 20% compared with 27%. In fact mothers having a caesarian delivery under epidural were no more likely than other mothers to stop breast feeding within two weeks; 20% compared with 19%. It therefore seems that it is the general anaesthetic rather than the caesarian delivery *per se* which has most effect on stopping breast feeding early.

4.5 Delays in starting breast feeding

Both the 1975 and the 1980 surveys found that how soon the baby was first put to the breast was strongly associated with success or failure of breast feeding in the first two weeks. Mothers who initiated breast feeding in the first few hours were much more likely to continue breast feeding than those who had started breast feeding later.

Clearly serious problems at the birth may delay initial

contact between mother and baby and thus hinder the start of breast feeding. But the previous surveys showed that in many cases mothers did not put the baby to the breast until some time after they first held the baby. Table 4.5 and 4.6 show this still to be the case in 1985. Table 4.5 shows that in 1985 almost 80% of women who subsequently breast fed said they had held their baby immediately; an increase on the 63% who did so in 1980. However, Table 4.6 shows that only 27% of these mothers put their baby to the breast immediately, despite having had the opportunity to do so. Even within an hour of the birth only 59% of mothers had put the baby to the breast. However, Table 4.6 indicates that there has been an improvement since 1980 when only 16% of mothers put their baby to the breast immediately after the birth. Moreover, the proportion of mothers experiencing delays in starting breast feeding of more than four hours had fallen to 24% compared with 35% in 1980.

However, this improvement did not result in fewer mothers stopping breast feeding in the first two weeks, as Table 4.7 shows. Only 14% of mothers who started breast feeding within the first hour stopped breast feeding within two weeks – similar to the 1980 figure of 13%, whereas 24% of those who first breast fed at times between four and twelve hours after the birth gave up within two weeks, as did 21% in 1980. A delay of more than twelve hours in starting breast feeding was associated with a significantly increased likelihood of stopping breast feeding early; 31% of such mothers gave up within two weeks. However, delays of such length were generally because either the mother or baby had had problems. Most commonly the mother had had a difficult delivery and/or the baby had needed

Table 4.5 Length of time until mothers who breast fed first held their babies (1980 and 1985 Great Britain)

Time until mother held baby	1980	1985
	%	%
Immediately	63	79
Within an hour	24	9
More than 1 hour up to 12 hours later	9	9
More than 12 hours later	4	3
	100	100
Base:	*2,734*	*3,319*

Table 4.6 Length of time until baby was put to the breast (1980 and 1985 Great Britain)

Time until baby was put to the breast	1980	1985
	%	%
Immediately	16	27
Within an hour	30	32
More than 1 hour up to 4 hours later	19	17
More than 4 hours up to 12 hours later	20	14
More than 12 hours	15	10
	100	100
Base:	*2,734*	*3,319*

Table 4.7 Proportion of mothers who had stopped breast feeding within two weeks by the length of time until the baby was first put to the breast (1980 and 1985 Great Britain)

Time until baby was put to the breast	1980	1985	1980	1985
	Percentage stopping breast feeding within two weeks		*Bases:*	
Immediately	13	14	*423*	*869*
Within an hour	13	15	*799*	*1,011*
More than 1 hour up to 4 hours later	18	21	*500*	*553*
More than 4 hours up to 12 hours later	21	24	*564*	*446*
More than 12 hours later	32	31	*422*	*327*
Total*	19	19	*2,734*	*3,319*

* Includes some cases where time until baby was put to breast was not known

admission to special care. Although in general mothers were initiating breast feeding sooner after the birth in 1985 than in 1980, those experiencing delays of between one and twelve hours were somewhat more likely to stop breast feeding in the first two weeks than had been the case in 1980. These two changes counterbalance one another resulting in no net change in stopping breast feeding in the first two weeks.

4.6 Special care

Quite apart from the clinical condition of the baby, special baby care is likely to affect early contact between mother and baby, and hence delay the initiation of breast feeding. In 1985, 25% of babies received special care; the proportion among those that were breast fed initially was 21%, compared with 17% in 1980. As in 1980, 23% of mothers whose babies had had special care stopped breast feeding within two weeks – a higher proportion than among other mothers. However, Table 4.8 indicates that it is the delay in starting breast feeding associated with special care which seems to have the adverse effect on breast feeding. If breast feeding is started within 24 hours, special care appears to have little effect on breast feeding compared to the length of the delay in starting. For delays longer than 24 hours mothers whose babies did not receive special care were more likely to give up breast feeding than those who did, indicating that the mother rather than the baby was likely to have been ill.

Table 4.8 Proportion of mothers who had stopped breast feeding within two weeks by length of time until the baby was put to the breast and whether or not special care was received (1980 and 1985 Great Britain)

Time until baby was put to the breast	1980		1985	
	Special care	No special care	Special care	No special care
	Percentage stopping breast feeding within two weeks			
Within 12 hours	20	16	20	17
More than 12 hours, up to 24 hours	26	33	32	29
More than 24 hours	27	41	23	46
All babies*	23	18	23	18
Bases:				
Within 12 hours	256	2,019	454	2,347
More than 12 hours, up to 24 hours	63	134	58	74
More than 24 hours	139	86	123	60
All babies*	463	2,259	660	2,521

* Includes some cases where time until baby was put to breast was not known

4.7 Birthweight

Babies may receive special care for a number of reasons, particularly low birthweight or prematurity. The smallest and weakest babies need feeding by a drip or tube until they are strong enough to suck from the breast or the bottle. It is therefore not surprising that the previous surveys have found an association between low birthweight and stopping breast feeding within two weeks. Table 4.9 shows that this is still the case in 1985, and that there has been little change since 1980.

Table 4.9 Proportion of mothers who had stopped breast feeding within two weeks by baby's birthweight (1980 and 1985 Great Britain)

Birthweight	1980	1985	1980	1985
	Percentage stopping breast feeding within two weeks		Bases	
Less than 2,500g	27	24	146	168
2,500g–2,999g	22	20	504	556
3,000g–3,499g	18	19	1,087	1,281
3,500g or more	18	18	996	1,260
All breast fed babies*	19	19	2,734	3,319

* Includes some cases where birthweight was not known

4.8 Estimating the effect of events at the time of birth on stopping breast feeding within two weeks

The analysis presented so far in this chapter has shown that a number of events occurring during labour and delivery and soon after the birth are associated with mothers giving up breast feeding within two weeks. A similar picture has emerged to that based on the 1980 results. As in 1980 we next take into account the relationships between the variables examined so far to discover which have the most significant effect on breast feeding in the early weeks.

It has already been shown that it is the general anaesthetic rather than the caesarian delivery which seems to have most effect on stopping breast feeding, and thus only the former is considered in this analysis. We have also included whether or not breast feeding was initiated within four hours of the birth, whether the baby had special care or not and whether it was under 2,500g at birth. A similar analysis to that described in Chapter 2 was carried out. However, the results showed that once the effects of the other variables are taken into account, only delays in starting breast feeding of more than four hours had a significant effect on stopping in the first two weeks. Birthweight, special care and having a general anaesthetic only affected the likelihood of stopping breast feeding in the first two weeks by virtue of their association with delays in starting breast feeding.

4.9 Feeding schedules in hospital

Both previous surveys showed that mothers who breast fed on demand rather than at set feeding times while in hospital were less likely to stop breast feeding within two weeks. Moreover, the proportion of mothers reporting that they had to feed at set times declined significantly between the two previous surveys. By 1985 there had been a further decline: only 19% of breast feeding mothers reported having to feed at set times in hospital compared with 32% in 1980 (Table 4.10).

Table 4.10 Type of feeding schedule followed by breast feeding mothers in hospital (1980 and 1985 Great Britain)

Feeding schedule	1980	1985
	%	%
Set time	32	19
On demand	66	79
Some other arrangement	2	2
	100	100
Base:	2,703	3,281

Table 4.11 Proportion of mothers who had stopped breast feeding within two weeks by hospital feeding schedule (1980 and 1985 Great Britain)

Feeding schedule	1980	1985	1980	1985
	Percentage stopping breast feeding within two weeks		Bases:	
Set time	28	32	867	589
More flexible arrangement	16	17	1,798	2,635
All babies born in hospital	19	20	2,703	3,281

Table 4.11 shows that mothers who fed at set times were rather more likely than their counterparts in 1980 to stop breast feeding within two weeks: 32% compared with 28% in 1980. In both 1980 and 1985 similar, and significantly smaller proportions of those who had experienced a more flexible feeding schedule than those on fixed schedules stopped within this period of time. It may well be that advice on adopting fixed feeding schedules is given in conjunction with inappropriate advice generally and that it is this advice rather than merely following a fixed feeding schedule *per se* that is associated with the early stopping of breast feeding. However, it still appears important to encourage mothers to breast feed on demand from the start in order to help establish breast feeding.

4.10 Contact between mother and baby in hospital

Clearly it is easier for a mother to breast feed on demand if her baby is always by her side, but it is sometimes thought advisable for newborn babies to be kept in a separate nursery for at least part of the time in hospital in order to allow the mother to sleep without interruptions. However, this practice had declined significantly since 1980. As Table 4.12 shows, in 1985 47% of breast feeding mothers said that their baby was with them continuously while in hospital compared with only 17% in 1980. In 1985 a further 18% said that although the baby was sometimes away from them, they always fed the baby themselves, while only 26% said the nurses sometimes fed the baby. (The remaining 9% was accounted for by babies in special care.) This question was phrased somewhat differently in 1980 and so further comparisons are not possible.

Table 4.12 Contact between breast feeding mothers and babies while in hospital (1980 and 1985 Great Britain)

	1980	1985
	%	%
Mother and baby together continuously	17	47
Baby away sometimes –		
mother always feeds it	..⎱77	18⎱44
nurses sometimes feed it	..⎰	26⎰
Baby in incubator or special care most of the time	6	9
	100	100
Base:	2,703	3,281

4.11 Giving bottles to breast fed babies

Supplementing breast feeding with infant formula may be necessary for some babies who are underweight or unwell. Both the previous surveys found that it was common practice for breast fed babies to be given bottles of infant formula in hospital, and the 1980 survey showed a strong association between giving bottles of formula and stopping breast feeding in the first two weeks. Although we cannot show that giving bottles of infant formula to breast fed babies has a causal relationship with stopping breast feeding in the early weeks, on physiological grounds it would seem likely to interfere with the initiation of lactation, and it seems unlikely to be necessary on nutritional grounds for more than a small minority of babies.

Table 4.13 shows that there has been very little change since 1980 in the prevalence of giving bottles of infant formula to breast fed babies: almost half had received some in the first week of life, although in most cases this was not on a regular basis. Table 4.14 shows that as in 1980 there is a significant association with stopping breast feeding in the first two weeks: only 8% of mothers whose babies had not received any infant formula stopped within this time compared with 28% of those whose babies had. For the minority of babies who had received infant formula at most feeds there was an even stronger relationship, but this may be because the mothers were having problems with breast feeding and were intending to give up. It is thus not possible from surveys such as these to examine fully the causal relationships involved, but it would seem advisable to follow the recommendations in *Present day practice in infant feeding: third report*[5] and to avoid giving infant formula to breast fed babies as far as possible.

Table 4.13 Frequency with which bottle of formula milk were given to breast fed babies in the first week (1980 and 1985 Great Britain)

	First births	
	1980	1985
	%	%
No bottles given	49	48
Mother uncertain whether bottles given	2	2
Bottles given once or twice only*	23	22
Bottles given during the night	9	9
Bottles given at every feed	11	9
Changed to bottle feeding completely by end of week†	3	–
Bottles given – other arrangement	2	7
Bottle given, mother not sure how often	1	1
	100	100
Base:	2,734	3,281

* *In 1980 this category included 'up to three bottles in first week' and 'bottles given where necessary'*
† *Not asked for in 1985*

Table 4.14 Proportion of mothers who had stopped breast feeding within two weeks by frequency with which bottles of milk had been given in the first week (1980 and 1985 Great Britain)

	1980	1985	1980	1985
	Percentage stopping breast feeding within two weeks		Bases:	
No bottles given	7	8	1,312	1,544
Bottles given occasionally or at night	16	20	925	997
Bottles given at most feeds	65	57	295	301
All babies who received a bottle while being breast fed*	31	28	1,313	1,606
All breast fed babies†	19	20	2,703	3,281

* *Bases do not add to total as some mothers failed to say how often their baby had received a bottle*
† *Does not include home births*

4.12 Combined effect of feeding schedules, giving infant formula and delays in starting breast feeding

The previous few sections have shown associations between a number of events occurring in hospital and stopping breast feeding in the first two weeks. Table 4.15 shows the effect of three of these in combination: whether the baby was given bottles of infant formula in the first week, whether the mother fed the baby at set times or according to a more flexible feeding schedule and whether she started breast feeding within four hours of the birth. Each cell of the table shows the proportion of mothers who stopped breast feeding within two weeks for the eight possible combinations of the three variables.

Table 4.15 Proportion of mothers who had stopped breast feeding within two weeks by whether bottles of infant formula were given, type of feeding schedule followed and length of time until baby was put to the breast (1985 Great Britain)

Time until baby was put to the breast/feeding schedule in hospital	Whether bottles of infant formula were given in the first week			
	Bottles given	No bottles given	*Bottles given*	*No bottles given*
	Percentage stopping breast feeding within two weeks		*Bases:*	
Four hours or less				
Flexible	24	7	*874*	*1,214*
Set times	34	16	*184*	*150*
Over four hours				
Flexible	30	18	*363*	*222*
Set times	38	34	*186*	*87*

The largest differences were between those whose babies received bottles of infant formula and those who did not: for each of the four combinations of the other two variables there were significant differences according to whether the babies had received infant formula. Among those mothers whose babies had not received any infant formula in the first week, delays in starting breast feeding and the type of feeding schedule adopted were each significantly and independently associated with stopping breast feeding in the first two weeks. However, these relationships were much less marked among mothers whose babies had received infant formula, although the type of feeding schedule was more important than whether delays in starting breast feeding had occurred. Again, the interpretation of these results is not straightforward: in particular delays in starting breast feeding and the need to give infant formula may be the result of other problems rather than the cause of breast feeding problems. Only a longitudinal study rather than retrospectively collected survey information can adequately investigate the causal relationships.

4.13 Feeding problems in hospital

Feeding problems while still in hospital were reported by 30% of breast feeding mothers, and not surprisingly were more common among mothers of first babies, 39% of whom reported problems compared with 21% of mothers of second and subsequent babies. Table 4.16 shows the types of problems they experienced. The mother having sore or cracked nipples was the most common problem experienced, and problems with the baby not latching on to the breast properly also featured strongly. These two problems are probably related, as it is thought by many experts that sore nipples result when the baby is incorrectly positioned and cannot latch on properly. It is important that adequate help is available for new mothers to teach them how the baby should be positioned and to check that this is done correctly, since problems may not become apparent until after the mother has left hospital. A mother reporting the problem of the baby being hungry presumably meant that the baby was crying with what appeared to be hunger. Although this is clearly distressing, mothers can be encouraged to see this as a short term problem which can be overcome by more frequent feeding to increase the supply of milk rather than a reason to abandon breast feeding.

Mothers were asked whether while they were in hospital they were always able to get help or advice when they needed it. The overwhelming majority said that they could: 64% of breast feeding mothers said that help was always available and 31% said it was generally available. Only 5% said this was not the case.

Table 4.16 Feeding problems experienced by breast feeding mothers while in hospital (1985 Great Britain)

	First births	Later births	All babies
	%	%	%
Had problems	39	21	30
Did not have problems	61	79	70
Base:	*1,612*	*1,643*	*3,254*

Problems experienced by those who had problems:

	Percentage having problem		
Sore/cracked nipples	27	30	28
Baby not latching on to breast	24	14	20
Baby hungry	19	19	19
Baby ill	14	16	15
Baby did not like milk	8	10	9
Baby vomiting	2	6	4
Baby got to much/ too little wind	1	3	2
Baby constipated	–	0	0
Other	23	18	21
Base:	*628*	*342*	*970*

Percentages do not add up to 100 as some mothers experienced more than one type of feeding problem

4.14 Breast feeding at home

Most mothers stay in hospital for only a few days and therefore do not have the opportunity to establish breast feeding properly before they return home. Although most have a daily visit from a midwife, in general there is less help available than when they were in hospital. They may also have more demands on them in terms of domestic chores and the care of older children which, together with the inevitable interrupted night's sleep, can make it difficult to cope with the demands of breast feeding. We therefore asked about the problems experienced at this time and looked at how many mothers had given up breast feeding by six weeks.

As reported at the beginning of the chapter, of those mothers who started breast feeding 15% had given up before they left hospital and a further 12% were giving bottles as well as breast feeding when they were discharged. Of those who were breast feeding at all when they left hospital 30% had given up by six weeks. Not surprisingly, those who were giving bottles as well as breast feeding when they left hospital were very much more likely to have stopped by six weeks than those who were breast feeding exclusively: 64% of the former compared with 24% of the latter.

Of mothers who were breast feeding when they left hospital, 34% said they had experienced problems with feeding their babies after they returned home. Mothers of first babies were more likely than mothers of later babies to report problems: 36% compared with 32%. Table 4.17 shows the problems they reported. By far the most common problem was the baby was thought to be hungry. As we showed at the beginning of the chapter this was the main reason given by mothers for stopping breast feeding at this stage. There may be times when a mother has less milk, particularly if she is tired or anxious, or the baby's appetite increases. Mothers need to be aware that this is a very common problem and it is not necessarily permanent. Mothers were asked whether they fed their baby on demand or kept to set feeding times when they returned home. Only a minority said they kept to set times (21%), but they were much more likely than those who fed on demand to have given up breast feeding by six weeks – 49% compared with 23%.

Mothers who experienced problems were more likely than other mothers to give up breast feeding by six weeks, as Table 4.18 shows. Once a mother is back at home informed advice is not always available so it is important that mothers are forewarned of the common problems with breast feeding in the early weeks and how they may be prevented or overcome without the mothers giving up breast feeding. Mothers who had experienced problems with breast feeding when they returned home were asked whether they had received any help; the vast majority (93%) had. The main source of advice was a health visitor (63%), followed by a midwife (46%) and a doctor (26%). Other people, such as friends or relatives were only cited as a source of help by 18%, which may reflect the lack of people with experience of successful breast feeding available to help new mothers.

Table 4.17 Feeding problems experienced by breast feeding mothers after leaving hospital (1985 Great Britain)

	First births	Later births	All babies
	%	%	%
Had problems	36	32	34
Did not have problems	64	68	66
Base:	*1,298*	*1,448*	*2,746*

Problems experienced by those who had problems:

	Percentage having problem		
Sore/cracked nipples	19	25	22
Baby not latching on to breast	5	3	4
Baby hungry	52	48	50
Baby ill	5	7	6
Baby did not like milk	8	4	6
Baby vomiting	6	7	7
Baby got too much/ too little wind	8	11	10
Baby constipated	3	2	3
Other	15	17	16
Base:	*457*	*447*	*904*

Percentages do not add up to 100 as some mothers experienced more than one type of feeding problem

Table 4.18 Proportion of mothers who had stopped breast feeding between leaving hospital and six weeks by whether they experienced feeding problems at home and birth order (1985 Great Britain)

	First births	Later births	All births	First births	Later births	All births
	Percentage stopping breast feeding by six weeks			*Bases:*		
Whether experienced feeding problems at home						
Yes	46	40	43	*468*	*461*	*929*
No	24	22	23	*830*	*987*	*1,817*
Whether those who had problems were given help	%	%	%			
Yes	94	92	93			
No	6	8	7			
	100	100	100			

5 Infant formula and bottle feeding

5.1 Introduction

In 1985 36% of mothers gave infant formula feeds from birth. Of those who started breast feeding 39% had stopped by six weeks and some of those who continued were giving formula as well as breast feeds. Thus by the time they were four weeks old the majority of babies in Great Britain were being fed infant formulas and at four months three quarters of babies were fully bottle fed. It is clearly important that mothers should know how to prepare and give infant formula feeds as well as knowing how to breast feed.

This chapter first defines the various types of infant formulas and then goes on to look at both the use of infant formula and of liquid cow's milk together with some of the problems experienced by mothers who were bottle feeding.

When looking at the use of infant formula beyond the age of about six weeks, that is after the first stage questionnaire had been completed, we have excluded from the analyses any mothers who ever used any of the 'Ostermilk' brands. This is because these infant formulas were withdrawn from the market just before the time when the second stage questionnaire was sent out.

5.2 Definition of infant formula

Infant formulas are artificial feeds which are manufactured to take the place of human milk. The manufacture process used is designed to make the composition of the final product as close to, and as biologically adequate as human milk. Most brands of infant formula can be classified into one of two types; either whey dominant or casein dominant, depending on whether whey or casein is the dominant protein. Whey dominant infant formulas have a whey:casein ratio which is closer to that in human milk whereas casein dominant formulas have a whey:casein ratio which is closer to that in cow's milk. Some manufacturers claim that a baby may be more satisfied by a casein dominant formula than by a whey dominant one, although there is no firm evidence to show that one type of infant formula is more suitable than the other. However when a mother is choosing which type to give her baby she may well be influenced by such claims from manufacturers.

The majority of infant formulas which are at present available in Great Britain are based on cow's milk but some formulas contain other proteins, for example soya protein.

'Follow-up milks' are artificial foods intended to constitute the milk element in the more diversified diets of babies over four months old. They contain more iron and vitamin D and less saturated fatty acids than whole cow's milk.

5.3 Additional bottles of milk

Mothers who breast feed may, in addition, give their babies bottles of infant formula. For those who were still breast feeding at the time of completing the first questionnaire, when the babies were about six weeks old, Table 5.1 shows whether bottles were also being given. The same table also shows the position at four months. Mothers were not asked details about when they gave bottles so we do not know whether they were giving them with breast milk at the same feed, or at a different feed. It is clear from the table that in 1985 breast fed babies were more likely to be receiving bottles in addition to breast milk, than in 1980. In 1985 a third of babies who were breast fed at six weeks were also receiving bottles compared with just over a quarter in 1980. Similarly at four months almost a quarter were receiving bottles compared with a fifth in 1980.

Table 5.1 Bottles given to breast fed babies at about six weeks and four months (1980 and 1985 Great Britain)

	Age of baby			
	About six weeks		About four months	
	1980	1985	1980	1985
	%	%	%	%
No bottles given	72	66	81	76
Bottles given	28	34	19	24
	100	100	100	100
Base: breast fed babies	*1,520*	*1,720*	*1,021**	*1,192**

* Bases are the reweighted numbers

Thus although there was little change between 1980 and 1985 in either the incidence or the duration of breast feeding, it appears that bottle feeding was more widespread in 1985 as more breast fed babies were also being given bottle feeds.

5.4 The use of non-human milk at different ages

Information was collected at all three stages about the type of non-human milk being given to babies. Table 5.2 shows the results for each stage for mothers who were bottle feeding at that stage and Table 5.3 shows the results separately for mothers who were bottle feeding exclusively and for mothers who were also breast feeding.

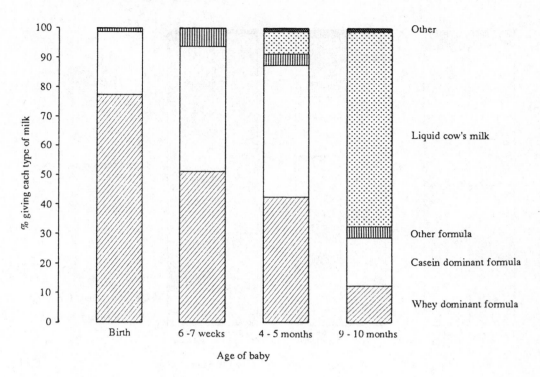

Figure 5.1   Main type of non-human milk given at each stage by mothers who were bottle feedin
(1985 Great Britain)

Table 5.2 Main type of non-human milk given at each stage by mothers who were bottle feeding (1985 Great Britain)

Type of non-human milk	Mothers bottle feeding at:			
	Birth	Stage 1 (6–7 weeks)	Stage 2 (4–5 months)	Stage 3 (9–10 months)
	%	%	%	%
Whey dominant	78	50	43	12
Casein dominant	21	43	46	16
Other formula eg soya based, 'follow-up milk'	1	6	4	4
Liquid cow's milk:	–	0	7	67
Whole	–	0	6	60
Semi-skimmed	–	–	1	5
Skimmed	–	–	0	2
Other/vague	–	–	1	1
Total	100	100	100	100
Base:	1,903	4,072	4,313*	5,048*

* Bases are the reweighted numbers

5.4.1 The use of infant formulas at different ages

Figure 5.1 and Table 5.2 show that there is a clear trend away from using whey dominant infant formulas as the baby gets older. At birth 78% of mothers giving any non-human milk were giving a whey dominant infant formula whereas at stage 2 only 43% were doing so. The use of casein dominant infant formulas increased sharply from 21% at birth to 43% at stage 1. Between stages 1 and 2 the use of casein dominant formulas stayed fairly constant, but decreased to 16% at stage 3 as mothers were increasingly using liquid cow's milk.

About 3% of mothers were giving a soya dominant formula at each stage, two mothers were giving a 'follow-up milk' at stage 1 and 1% were doing so at stages 2 and 3. Only a very small proportion of mothers who

had given a 'follow-up milk' had done so before the baby was four months old; the majority did not do so before the baby was six months old.

Figure 5.2 and Table 5.3 compare the use of non-human milk by mothers bottle feeding exclusively at each stage with that by mothers who were also breast feeding. It is noticeable that at both stages 1 and 2 mothers who were also breast feeding were very much more likely to be giving a whey dominant than a casein dominant infant formula. At stages 2 and 3 these mothers were also more likely to be giving liquid cow's milk than those who were exclusively bottle feeding and they were also more likely to be giving some other type of formula, which was usually a soya dominant one.

Figure 5.2 Comparison of main type of non-human milk given at each stage between mothers who were bottle feeding exclusively and those who were also breast feeding (1985 Great Britain)

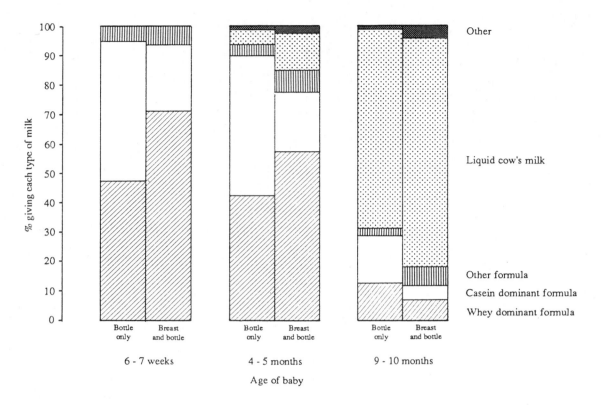

Table 5.3 Main type of non-human milk given at each stage by mothers who were bottle feeding exclusively and mothers who were also breast feeding (1985 Great Britain)

Type of non-human milk	Mothers bottle feeding exclusively at:				Mothers who were also breast feeding at:		
	Birth	Stage 1 (6–7 weeks)	Stage 2 (4–5 months)	Stage 3 (9–10 months)	Stage 1 (6–7 weeks)	Stage 2 (4–5 months)	Stage 3 (9–10 months)
	%	%	%	%	%	%	%
Whey dominant	78	47	42	13	70	58	7
Casein dominant	21	46	47	16	23	20	5
Other formula eg soya based, 'follow-up milk'	1	5	4	3	6	8	6
Liquid cow's milk:							
Whole	–	0	5	67	0	12	78
	–	0	5	59	0	11	67
Semi-skimmed	–	–	0	5	–	2	8
Skimmed	–	–	0	2	–	0	3
Other/vague	–	–	1	1	–	3	4
Total	100	100	100	100	100	100	100
Base:	*1,903*	*3,503*	*4,031**	*4,758**	*569*	*282**	*290**

* Bases are the reweighted numbers

In order to get a better idea of the pattern of milk usage followed by bottle feeding mothers in the early weeks, Tables 5.4 and 5.5 show the use of whey and casein dominant formulas at different ages separately for those mothers who bottle fed from birth and for those mothers who breast fed initially. Mothers who had ever used any of the Ostermilks have been excluded from Tables 5.4 and 5.5 as they may have stopped using these milks for reasons beyond their control.

Table 5.4 shows much the same pattern as Figure 5.1, that there is a clear trend away from using whey dominant formulas as the baby gets older and that the use of casein dominant formulas increases in the first ten weeks or so and then falls off as mothers start to use other milks, mainly cow's milk.

Table 5.4 The use of whey and casein dominant infant formulas at different stages by those who bottle fed from birth (1985 Great Britain)

	Birth	Stage 1 (6–7 weeks)	Stage 2 (4–5 months)	Stage 3 (9–10 months)
	%	%	%	%
Whey dominant	79	51	41	15
Casein dominant	20	48	49	20
Other	1	1	10	65
	100	100	100	100
Base:	*1,219*	*1,219*	*1,219*	*1,219*

For mothers of babies who were initially breast fed the same trend is apparent (Table 5.5). The younger the baby was the more likely it was that he or she was given a whey dominant formula. The use of casein dominant

Table 5.5 First infant formula given to babies who were initially breast fed by baby's age when breast feeding ceased (1985 Great Britain)

	Baby's age when breast feeding ceased:			
	Less than 1 week	1 week but less than 2 weeks	2 weeks but less than 2 months	2 months or more
	%	%	%	%
Whey dominant	86	79	77	67
Casein dominant	13	18	21	22
Other	1	3	2	11
	100	100	100	100
Base:	285	106	554	811*

* Bases are the reweighted numbers

formulas went up from 13% for babies of less than one week old to 21% of babies aged between two weeks and two months but after this there was little increase as mothers introduced other milks.

5.4.2 Choice of type of infant formula

It seems from the above analyses that mothers who bottle feed first give their baby a whey dominant formula and as the baby gets older switch to a casein dominant formula. In order to look in more detail at whether mothers choose whey or casein dominant formulas this section looks at the changes made by individual mothers in the type of formula they used. On the first stage questionnaire mothers were asked whether they had changed from using one infant formula to another, and if so why they had stopped using the first one. Of just over 4,000 mothers who were bottle feeding at six to ten weeks, 44% had changed the type of infant formula they were giving by six to ten weeks and a minority of these mothers had changed more than

Table 5.6 Changes between whey dominant and casein dominant infant formulas in the first 6–10 weeks (1985 Great Britain)

Type of change of infant formula given	Number of changes			
	1	2	3	All changes
	%	%	%	%
Whey to whey	20	4	9	16
Whey to casein	64	28	22	54
Casein to whey	7	19	11	10
Casein to casein	5	43	43	15
Other	4	6	15	5
	100	100	100	100
Base: number of changes	1,799	566	151	2,427*

* Including 27 fourth changes

once. The formulas used were classified according to whether the dominant protein was whey, casein or other, and the types of changes made were examined. Table 5.6 shows that the most common first change was from a whey to a casein dominant infant formula, 64% of first changes, with a change from one whey dominant to another also being quite common, 20%. For subsequent changes a change from one casein dominant brand to another was the most frequent type of change.

Table 5.7 shows that the most common reason for changing the type of infant formula was because the mother thought the baby was still hungry or not satisfied. This reason was given for over two thirds of the changes made. It was by far the most common reason given for changing from a whey to a casein dominant formula and also for changing between casein dominant formulas. It seems that mothers turn from a whey to a casein dominant formula because they feel that the baby is still hungry after a feed and then if they make another change it is to another casein dominant brand, again because they feel that the baby is still hungry. Although allergy was not frequently mentioned as a reason for changing brands it was particularly associated with 'other' changes, which were usually to a soya dominant formula.

The majority of mothers who had changed the brand of infant formula they were using by six to ten weeks had been advised to do so. Table 5.8 shows that 29% had

Table 5.8 Sources of advice on changing milk brands in the first 6–10 weeks by birth order (1985 Great Britain)

Source of advice	First births	Later births	All babies
	Percentage receiving advice		
No one	22	35	29
Health visitor	42	41	42
Midwife or nurse	19	18	19
Friend or relative	20	7	14
Doctor	7	6	7
Other	1	1	19
Base:	881	908	1,788

Percentages do not add up to 100 as some mothers were advised to change milks by more than one source

changed the brand of infant formula on their own initiative. The person most likely to have advised mothers to change brands was the health visitor; 42% had received advice from her. Mothers of first babies were less likely than mothers of later babies to have changed brands without anyone advising them to, and they were more likely to have been advised by a friend or relative.

Table 5.7 Reasons given by mother for changing between whey dominant and casein dominant infant formula (1985 Great Britain)

Reason	Whey to whey	Whey to casein	Casein to whey	Casein to casein	Other change	All changes
	Percentage giving reason					
Still hungry/not satisfied	41	85	46	71	15	69
Kept being sick	32	11	30	18	28	18
Constipation	15	7	21	14	5	10
Allergy	1	1	3	3	33	3
Other reason	22	5	17	7	29	10
Base: number of changes	392	1,301	245	374	115	2,427

* Percentages do not add up to 100 as some mothers gave more than one reason for a particular change

5.4.3 The use of liquid cow's milk

As Table 5.2 and Figure 5.1 have shown, less than 1% of mothers who were giving any non-human milk were giving their babies liquid cow's milk at the time the first questionnaire was completed. By the second stage this figure had risen to 5%, and by the third stage 67% were giving it. Thus by the time the baby was 9–10 months old liquid cow's milk had become the predominant milk.

On the third stage questionnaire mothers were asked what type of milk they were giving as the main milk, as a second milk and to mix solid food. Table 5.9 shows that by the time the babies were 9–10 months old 88% of all mothers were giving their baby liquid cow's milk in some way. The most common usage of liquid cow's milk at this age was to mix food (78%), next came giving it as the main milk (64%) and relatively few mothers were giving it as the second milk (15%).

Table 5.9 Liquid cow's milk given at stage 3 (9–10 months) (1985 Great Britain)

Proportion of mothers who gave liquid cow's milk	
As main milk:	64
Whole	57
Semi-skimmed	5
Skimmed	2
As second milk:	15
Whole	11
Semi-skimmed	3
Skimmed	1
To mix food	78
All using liquid cow's milk	88
Base:	*5,223**

Percentages do not add up to 100 as some mothers gave liquid cow's milk in more than one way
* Base is the reweighted number

The vast majority of mothers who were giving their babies liquid cow's milk were giving whole cow's milk. However 11% of those giving cow's milk as the main milk and 27% of those giving it as a second milk were giving either semi-skimmed or skimmed milk. This is rather worrying as it is recommended in *Present day practice in infant feeding: third report*[5] that fully skimmed and semi-skimmed milks are not suitable for an infant's diet.

At both stages 2 and 3 mothers were asked at what age they had first given the milks they were currently using, either as a drink or to mix solid food. Thus we can examine the age at which liquid cow's milk is first introduced into the young child's diet. Figure 5.3 shows the earliest age at which liquid cow's milk was given at all, and one can see from this that in most cases it was not until the baby was over six months old that liquid cow's milk had been introduced. Table 5.10 shows the earliest age at which liquid cow's milk was given for the three types of usage: to mix solid food, as a main drink and as a second drink. Only 16% of mothers had given liquid cow's milk before the baby was five months old; this was generally to mix solid food rather than as a drink. Only 4% of mothers had given liquid cow's milk

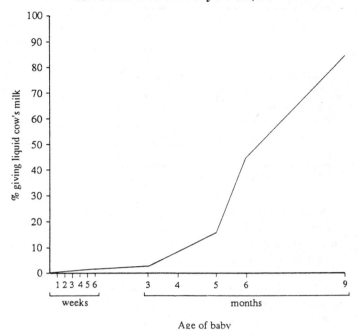

Figure 5.3 Age by which mothers had introduced liquid cow's milk into the baby's diet (1985 Great Britain)

as the main drink before five months, and the majority had not done so until the baby was at least six months old.

Table 5.10 Age by which mothers had introduced liquid cow's milk to mix solid food, as a main drink, or as a second drink (1985 Great Britain)

	Proportion of mothers who gave liquid cow's milk:			
	To mix food	As main drink	As second drink	At all
Before 6 weeks	1	0	0	1
Before 3 months	3	1	0	3
Before 4 months	8	2	0	9
Before 5 months	14	4	1	16
Before 6 months	39	23	3	45
Before 9 months	74	59	12	84
Base:	5,223	5,223	5,223	5,223

5.5 Problems with bottle feeding in hospital

Mothers who bottle feed as well as those who breast feed can experience problems feeding their baby in the early weeks. As the majority of mothers will give their baby infant formula at some stage it is important that all mothers, regardless of how they intend to feed their baby, should know how to make up a bottle of infant formula so as to minimise possible feeding problems. The 1985 survey found no significant difference in the proportions of mothers who had been taught how to make up a bottle in antenatal classes according to their planned feeding method. Seventy-two per cent of those intending to bottle feed, compared with 68% of those intending to breast feed, had received such tuition.

Bottle feeding mothers were less likely than breast feeding mothers to have experienced problems feeding their baby while in hospital. Even so 16% did have problems and not surprisingly mothers of first babies were more likely than other mothers to have had such problems, 18% compared with 14%. Table 5.11 shows the feeding problems that bottle feeding mothers had. The most common problems mentioned were the baby being ill and the baby being sick. Mothers experienced much the same sorts of problems regardless of whether it was their first baby or not. When asked whether while they were in hospital they were able to get help and advice when they needed it, almost all bottle feeding mothers said that they were; 69% said they were always able to, 27% said they were generally able to, and only 4% said that they were not able to.

Table 5.11 Feeding problems experienced by bottle feeding mothers while in hospital by birth order (1985 Great Britain)

Problem	First births	Later births	All babies
	Percentage having problem		
Baby hungry	17	13	15
Baby ill	31	33	32
Baby did not like milk	12	12	12
Baby vomiting	23	26	25
Baby got too much/ too little wind	9	5	7
Baby constipated	0	2	1
Other	21	21	21
Base:	*129*	*165*	*294*

Percentages do not add up to 100 as some mothers experienced more than one type of feeding problem

5.6 Free sample of infant formula

Some maternity units choose to give a small quantity of infant formula free to mothers who are leaving hospital so that they have an emergency supply in case they get into difficulties when they get home. Fifty-nine per cent of mothers who were bottle feeding on discharge, 58% of those who were giving both breast and bottle and 25% of those who were breast feeding only, were given infant formula to take home. The practice of giving samples of infant formula to mothers who are breast feeding goes against the principles of the International Code of Marketing of Breast-Milk Substitutes (WHO code).[6] There was no evidence from this survey, however, that breast feeding mothers who received a free sample of infant formula gave up breast feeding any sooner than those who did not.

Whether or not breast feeding mothers received infant formula was related to the region in which they had their baby. Table 5.12 shows that as one moves north the more likely mothers were to have received a free sample of infant formula.

Table 5.12 Proportion of mothers who were breast feeding on discharge from hospital who received a free sample of infant formula by region (1985 Great Britain)

		Bases:
London and the South East	20	*915*
South West and Wales	19	*351*
Midlands and East Anglia	28	*409*
North	32	*517*
Scotland	34	*197*
All regions	25	*2,392*

5.7 Problems with bottle feeding at home

Of those mothers who were bottle feeding when they left hospital, 22% experienced some problems feeding

their baby after they had returned home. Table 5.13 shows the problems that these mothers had. By far the most common problem now that the babies were a bit older was the baby being hungry, the most common problem experienced by breast feeders as well. All mothers need to be aware that a baby crying with what appears to be hunger is a very common problem. Again the sorts of problems experienced by bottle feeding mothers were similar regardless of birth order.

The vast majority of mothers who had problems with bottle feeding received some sort of professional help or advice with these problems. Now that they had left hospital, the most likely person to have advised mothers on such matters was the health visitor; 63% of mothers said that they had been helped or advised by her.

Table 5.13 Feeding problems experienced by bottle feeding mothers after leaving hospital by birth order (1985 Great Britain)

Problem	First births	Later births	All babies
	Percentage having problem		
Baby hungry	45	41	43
Baby ill	11	14	12
Baby did not like milk	10	8	9
Baby vomiting	17	21	19
Baby got too much/ too little wind	17	16	17
Baby constipated	7	6	6
Other	10	14	12
Base:	*278*	*336*	*614*

Percentages do not add up to 100 as some mothers experienced more than one type of feeding problem

5.8 Information given on the labels of infant formula

Infant formulas are manufactured so that they are either liquids which are ready to feed, or liquids or powders that require the addition only of water and no other substance. Detailed instructions about the preparation of feeds is clearly set out by manufacturers on the labels of their packs. On the stage 2 questionnaire, when the babies were aged between four and five months, mothers who were bottle feeding were asked whether they ever read the labels on tins or packets of infant formula. Fifty-six per cent said that they usually read the label, 34% said that they sometimes did and 10% said that they never did. Mothers of first babies were no more likely to have read these labels than other mothers, but mothers in the higher social classes were more likely to have read these labels than those in the lower social classes or those who had no husband or partner (Table 5.14). Whether or not a mother read the label was also related to her education, those who left school after the age of 18 were most likely to have read the label (Table 5.15).

On the whole mothers found the information on the labels easy to understand. Thirty-five per cent thought it was very easy to understand, 51% thought it was quite easy, 12% thought it was quite difficult and 2% thought it was very difficult. The majority of mothers, 84%, also found the information helpful, mothers of first babies more so than other mothers, 86% compared with 83%.

Table 5.14 Whether or not mother reads labels on tins or packets of infant formula by social class (1985 Great Britain)

	Social class								
	I	II	IIINM	IIIM	IV	V	Unclassified	No partner	Total
	%	%	%	%	%	%	%	%	%
Yes – usually	67	64	57	53	52	49	56	53	56
Yes – sometimes	27	27	36	37	38	38	32	34	34
No – never	6	9	7	10	10	13	12	13	10
	100	100	100	100	100	100	100	100	100
Base:	188*	707*	348*	1,417*	664*	233*	144*	531*	4,232*

* Bases are the reweighted numbers

Table 5.15 Whether or not mother reads labels on tins or packets of infant formula by mother's age at finishing full-time education (1985 Great Britain)

	Mother's age at finishing full-time education			
	16 or under	17 or 18	Over 18	Total
	%	%	%	%
Yes – usually	52	59	66	56
Yes – sometimes	37	31	28	34
No – never	11	10	6	10
	100	100	100	100
Base:	2,686*	1,074*	449*	4,232†

* Bases are the reweighted numbers
† Includes some cases where mother's age at finishing full-time education was not known

Mothers were asked whether there were any changes they would like to see to the labels and Table 5.16 shows their replies. Over half the mothers, 59%, were quite satisfied with what was said already and did not want to see any changes. The change most often requested by mothers was for the label to contain the same information but to have it explained more clearly. Mothers were also asked if there was any additional information, apart from the contents, that they would like to see on the label. Again most mothers seemed satisfied with the current situation, only 16% said that they wanted any addition and the most popular of these was for more nutritional information to be included; however only 6% requested this.

Table 5.16 Changes that mothers would like to see on labels of packets or tins of infant formula by birth order (1985 Great Britain)

	First births	Later births	All babies
	Percentage wanting change		
None – satisfied with what is on the label	62	57	59
The same information but explained more clearly	28	33	31
The exact quantities of each ingredient	11	11	11
Something else	2	2	2
Base:	1,762*	1,995*	3,757*

* Bases are the reweighted numbers

5.9 Cost of milk for the baby

In 1985 all pregnant women and families with a child under five who were on supplementary benefit, or family income supplement, or whose income was low were entitled to tokens for free milk or infant formula. At each stage of the survey mothers were asked whether they got milk tokens and Table 5.17 shows the results. The proportions of mothers receiving tokens was about 30% at each stage. The majority of those receiving tokens did so for the baby, although about a third received tokens for older children. Not surprisingly receiving milk tokens was strongly related to social class with those in the lower social classes or with no partner being most likely to get them.

At stages 2 and 3 mothers who were bottle feeding were asked how much they spent per week on milk for their baby. Table 5.18 shows that when the babies were aged between four and five months, a time when their diet would mainly be infant formula, most mothers were spending between £3.00 and £4.00 a week. Mothers who receive tokens for infant formula are entitled to two tins per week which would cost about £3.70, this seems to be in line with what mothers are spending on average. By the time the babies were between nine and ten months old the amount spent on milk had fallen, most mothers were spending between £1.00 and £2.00. At this stage mothers' answers to how much they were spending on milk for the baby are likely to be less accurate as liquid cow's milk would be a large proportion of the baby's diet and it would be difficult to determine exactly how much was being spent on this milk for the baby compared with the rest of the family.

Table 5.17 Whether mothers received milk tokens at different stages (1985 Great Britain)

	Stage 1 (6–7 weeks)	Stage 2 (4–5 months)	Stage 3 (9–10 months)
	Percentage receiving tokens		
Yes for the baby	24	26	26
Yes for herself	4	3	2
Yes for older children	10 }31	10 }30	10 }28
Had applied for tokens	2	1	1
No, did not receive tokens	69	70	72
Base:	5,223	5,223*	5,223*

* Bases are the reweighted numbers
Percentages do not add up to 100 as some mothers received milk tokens for more than one person

Table 5.18 Amount spent per week on milk for the baby by mothers who were bottle feeding exclusively (1985 Great Britain)

Amount spent per week	Baby aged:	
	4–5 months	9–10 months
	%	%
Less than £1.00	10	14
£1.00–£2.00	10	48
£2.00–£3.00	8	19
£3.00–£4.00	50	14
£4.00–£5.00	9	2
£5.00–£6.00	7	2
Over £6.00	6	1
	100	100
Average amount spent per week	£3.30	£1.70
Base:	3,541*	4,200*

* Bases are the reweighted numbers

6 Solid food, vitamins and other drinks

6.1 Introduction

Present day practice in infant feeding: third report[5] states that very few infants will require solid food before the age of three months but the vast majority should be offered a mixed diet not later than the age of six months. This chapter discusses the age at which mothers introduced solid food, what sorts of solids they were giving to babies at different ages, what factors influenced them in their choice of solids and the use of additional drinks and vitamin supplements. It also goes on to look at some of the problems mothers faced once the baby had got a bit older.

6.2 Age at introduction of solid food

Between 1980 and 1985 there has not been a great deal of change in the age at which mothers introduce solid food to babies (Table 6.1 and Figure 6.1). This is in contrast to the major change observed between 1975 and 1980 when the proportion of mothers giving solid

food before the age of three months had fallen from 85% to 56%.

In 1985 mothers were a little less likely to have introduced solids before six weeks than they were in 1980, but they were significantly more likely to have introduced solids before their baby was three months old. In 1985, 62% of babies had been given solids by the time they were three months old compared with 56% in 1980. As in 1980 virtually all babies had been given solids by the time they were six months old. The most common age for introducing solids in 1980 was between three and four months, whereas in 1985 it was between eight weeks and three months. It is clear that many mothers are still starting solid foods earlier than is generally thought to be desirable.

Both the 1975 and the 1980 surveys found an association between the age at which solids were started and the method of feeding: mothers who bottle fed started solids earlier than those who breast fed. Table 6.2

Table 6.1 Proportion of babies who had been given solid food by different ages (1980 and 1985 Great Britain)

Baby aged:	1980	1985
	Percentage giving solid food	
4 weeks	4	3
6 weeks	14	11
8 weeks	24	24
3 months	56	62
4 months	89	90
6 months	98	99
9 months	99	100
Base:	*4,224*	*5,223*

Table 6.2 Proportion of babies who had been given solid food by six weeks according to method of feeding (1980 and 1985 Great Britain)

Method of feeding at six weeks	1980	1985	*1980*	*1985*
	Percentage giving solid food		*Bases:*	
Breast	4	4	*1,666*	*1,711*
Bottle	21	14	*2,487*	*3,483*
Total	14	11	*4,208*	*5,194*

Figure 6.1 Proportion of babies who had been given solid food by different ages (1980 and 1985 Great Britain)

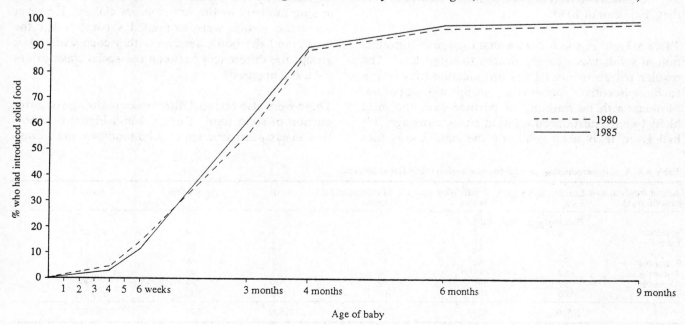

Table 6.3 Age at introduction of solid food by social class (1985 Great Britain)

Age at introduction of solid food	Social class								
	I	II	IIINM	IIIM	IV	V	Unclass-ified	No partner	Total
	Percentage giving solid food								
4 weeks	2	2	2	3	4	5	3	7	3
6 weeks	5	6	8	12	13	17	10	21	11
8 weeks	10	16	17	26	28	36	23	38	24
3 months	44	53	58	65	67	72	58	73	62
4 months	84	87	88	92	92	93	84	92	90
6 months	98	99	99	99	99	100	96	99	99
9 months	100	100	100	100	100	100	99	100	100
Base:	301	1,021	439	1,631	738	245	171	546	5,092

Figure 6.2 Age at introduction of solid food by social class (1985 Great Britain)

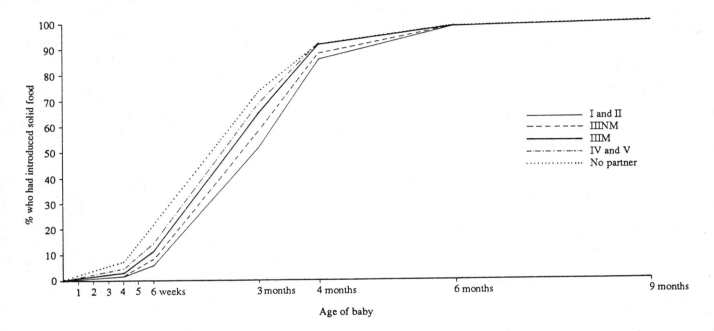

shows that this was still the case in 1985, 14% of mothers who were bottle feeding had given solid foods by six weeks compared with only 4% of mothers who were breast feeding. However bottle feeding mothers were less likely to have started solids by six weeks than they had been in 1980.

Table 6.3 and Figure 6.2 show that the age of introduction of solids was strongly related to social class. The regular pattern of an earlier introduction of solids in each consecutive social class group was apparent. Mothers with no husband or partner were the most likely to have introduced solids at a very early age, 7% had given their baby solids by the time it was four

weeks old and 73% had given solids by three months, the minimum recommended age for starting solids. In comparison only 44% of mothers in Social Class I had given solids by three months. These results might be explained by the higher prevalence of bottle feeding among mothers in the lower social classes. However when the results were examined separately for the breast and the bottle feeders within each social class group, the differences between the social class groups were still apparent.

There were also regional differences in the age of introduction of solid food. Table 6.4 and Figure 6.3 show that an early introduction of solid foods was more com-

Table 6.4 Age at introduction of solid food by region (1985 Great Britain)

Age at introduction of solid food	London and South East	South West and Wales	Midlands and East Anglia	North	Scotland	Total
	Percentage giving solid food					
4 weeks	2	3	5	3	6	3
6 weeks	7	11	13	13	18	11
8 weeks	16	25	27	27	32	24
3 months	55	61	67	67	64	62
4 months	87	89	90	93	90	90
6 months	99	99	98	99	99	99
9 months	100	100	100	100	100	100
Base:	1,580	655	978	1,340	539	5,092

Figure 6.3 Age at introduction of solid food by region (1985)

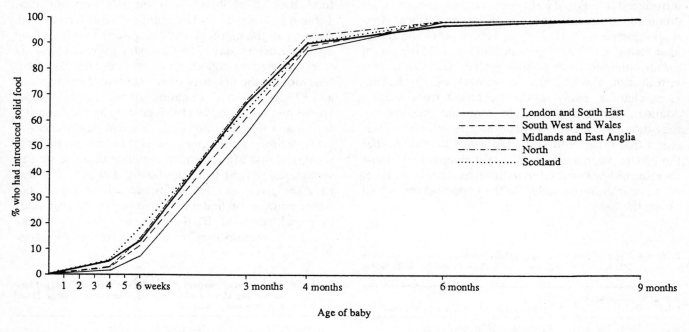

mon in Scotland than in London and the South East, with the other three regions falling in between. Again, even after allowing for the fact that mothers in the north were more likely than those in the south to be bottle feeding, the regional differences still held true.

Table 6.5 Age at introduction of solid food by smoking (1985 Great Britain)

Age at introduction of solid food	Smoking status during pregnancy:		
	Non-smoker	Smoker	Total
	Percentage giving solid food		
4 weeks	2	5	3
6 weeks	8	17	11
8 weeks	19	33	24
3 months	58	70	62
4 months	88	92	90
6 months	99	99	99
9 months	100	100	100
Base:	3,651	1,441	5,092

Mothers who smoked during pregnancy were more likely to have introduced solids earlier than those who did not (Table 6.5 and Figure 6.4). Seventy per cent of those who smoked, compared with 58% of those who did not, had introduced solids by three months. As we have already seen smoking is strongly related to social class, but within each social class group smokers had given solids earlier than non-smokers. This relationship also holds true if one looks at a mother's smoking behaviour before rather than during pregnancy.

Manufacturers of infant formulas have suggested that the use of a casein dominant formula will lead to a later introduction of solids. To examine this claim Table 6.6 looks at the type of infant formula each baby was being given just before solids were introduced and compares babies on casein dominant formulas with those on whey

Figure 6.4 Age at introduction of solid food by mother's smoking behaviour (1985 Great Britain)

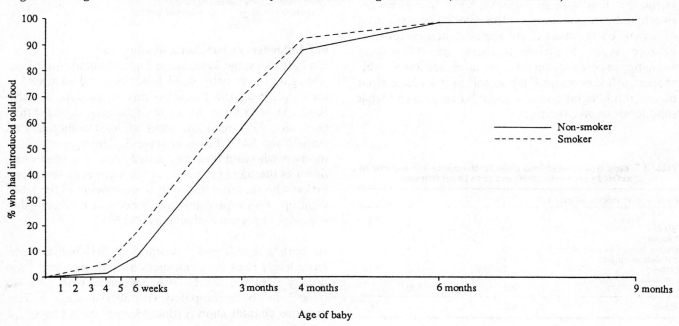

dominant formulas to see at what age each group was introduced to solids. Twenty per cent of babies on whey dominant formulas were given solids before eight weeks compared with 32% of babies on casein dominant formulas. Thus it does not appear that the use of casein dominant formulas necessarily leads to a later introduction of solid food. As we have seen in the previous chapter, many mothers changed from a whey dominant formula to a casein dominant one because they thought the baby was still hungry after a feed. It seems that if the baby still cried with what the mother thought to be hunger on a casein dominant formula then she either switched to a different casein dominant brand or introduced solids, in the hope that this would satisfy the baby.

Table 6.6 Type of infant formula babies were on before solids were introduced by age at introduction to solids (1985 Great Britain)

Age at introduction of solid food	Whey dominant	Casein dominant
	Percentage giving solid food	
4 weeks	2	5
6 weeks	9	16
8 weeks	20	32
3 months	60	73
4 months	90	95
6 months	99	99
9 months	100	100
Base:	*1,364*	*1,119*

6.3 Solid foods given at different ages

Mothers who had introduced solid food by the time the first questionnaire was completed were asked what they had given as the first solid food; their answers were classified into the five categories shown in Table 6.7. As in 1980 cereals and rusks were still by far the most common first solid foods for babies under six weeks old. Slightly fewer mothers had given rusks as the first food and slightly more had given cereal than had been the case in 1980. Of the mothers who had given cereal as the first food a large majority, 83%, had given unsweetened cereal. However, this may be because a lot of cereals on the market are unsweetened rather than because sugar conscious mothers are deliberately avoiding sweetened cereals. A later section in this chapter will shed more light on this as it looks at what factors mothers take into account when deciding what solid foods to give their baby.

Table 6.7 First type of solid food given by those who had introduced solids by six weeks (1980 and 1985 Great Britain)

First type of solid food given	1980	1985
	%	%
Rusk	56	52
Cereal	35	42
Dried, tinned or jars of food	4	3
Fresh/homemade	1	1
Other	4	2
	100	100
Base:	*605*	*559*

At all stages mothers were asked to list all the solid food their baby had eaten on the previous day. Table 6.8 shows the different foods mentioned at each stage by all the mothers who had given some solid food on the previous day. Mothers who gave solids at six weeks tended to choose rusks and cereals. By about four months the majority of mothers were giving solids and 82% of babies were eating commercial baby food. Home prepared foods were given only by the minority, the reason why was not clear. *Present day practice in infant feeding: third report*[5] states that 'there is much to commend first offering small amounts of home pureed vegetables or fruit from the family diet provided that they are given without additional salt or sugar', but some mothers will find it more convenient to give ready prepared babyfood. By the time the babies were aged about nine months they were being given a wide range of foods.

Table 6.8 Proportion of mothers who had given different kinds of food on one day at six weeks (stage 1), four months (stage 2) and at nine months (stage 3)

Type of food	Baby aged:		
	6 Weeks	4 Months	9 Months
	Percentage giving each food		
Cereal*	52	65	84
Rusk	54	40	28
Babyfood†	30	82	52
Homemade food**	3	35	
Other food**	2	8	
Yoghurt			26
Fresh fruit			26
Other dessert			21
Egg			21
Cheese			9
Meat			37
Fish			9
Potatoes			47
Other vegetables			49
Casserole/stew			12
Soup			7
Bread			64
Other foods			11
Base: all mothers who had given solid food	*1,299*	*4,930§*	*5,138§*

* Not known whether baby or adult cereal
† Commercially prepared tinned or dried food
§ Bases are the reweighted numbers
** Itemised in Stage 3 questionnaire only

6.4 Influences on the choice of solid food

On both the stage 2 and stage 3 questionnaires mothers who gave their baby solid food were asked whether they ever read the labels on tins or packets of baby food. At both these stages the vast majority said that they did; 93% read the label at least sometimes at stage 2 and 94% did so at stage 3. The proportion of mothers who said that they usually read the label went down as the baby got older, at the same time the proportion who said that they only sometimes read the label went up. This is probably a reflection of mothers gaining more experience of giving solid food.

At both stages 2 and 3 mothers of first babies were more likely than other mothers to have said that they usually read the label: 70% compared with 64% at stage 2 and 68% compared with 59% at stage 3. The previous chapter showed that whether or not mothers read the labels on infant formula was related to their social class and education. This was also the case with regard to reading the labels on babyfood. The vast majority of mothers found the information on the labels both easy to understand and helpful. At stage 2, 95% said that they thought the information was easy to understand and 94% found it helpful. These proportions remained the same at stage 3.

Mothers were asked whether there were any changes they would like to see on the labels of babyfood and Table 6.9 shows their replies. When the babies were aged 9–10 months mothers were less satisfied with the labels than they had been earlier. Twenty-eight per cent wanted the exact quantities of each ingredient included, and again, as was the case with the labels on infant formula, there was a plea to have the information explained more clearly – 26% wanted this. When asked if there was any additional information they would like to see on the label most mothers (82%) said there was not, although 9% of mothers said they would like to see more nutritional information.

Table 6.9 Changes that mothers would like to see on labels of packets or tins of babyfood at about four months (stage 2) and at nine months (stage 3) (1985 Great Britain)

	Baby aged:	
	4 months	9 months
	Percentage wanting change	
None – satisfied with what is on the label	61	49
The exact quantities of each ingredient	21	28
The same information but explained more clearly	20	26
Something else	5	7
Base:	4,656*	4,057*†

Percentages do not add up to 100 as some mothers wanted to see more than one change
* Bases are the reweighted numbers
† Excludes mothers who never gave commercial babyfood

In the second and the third stage questionnaires mothers were asked what they took into account when deciding what solid foods to give their baby. This was asked as an open question without any precodes or prompting and many mothers said they took several factors into account. The answers fell broadly into two groups: nutritional factors and non-nutritional factors, and are shown in Table 6.10. Some mention was made about general nutrition by 32% of mothers who were giving solid food at stage 2 and by 51% at stage 3. This included fairly unspecific comments like 'balanced diet', 'calories', 'what his digestion can cope with' or 'food value'. Sugar content was the next most common consideration with 29% of mothers mentioning this at stage 2 and 22% mentioning it at stage 3. Salt, vitamins and additives were mentioned by over 10% of mothers at each stage. Of the non-nutritional factors, variety was the most common thing mentioned. This included variety of tastes and textures, for example mothers liked foods that could be made up to different thicknesses or that the baby could chew.

Table 6.10 What mothers took account of when deciding what solid foods to give (1985 Great Britain)

	Baby aged:	
	4–5 months	9–10 months
	Percentage mentioning each factor	
Nutritional factors		
Nutrition generally eg 'balanced diet' 'food value'	32	51
Sugar content	29	22
Additives	14	18
Vitamins	13	14
Salt content	12	11
Gluten content	8	1
Protein content	5	8
Fat content	4	8
Mineral content	1	2
Carbohydrate content	1	2
Non-nutritional factors		
Variety	30	27
Baby's preferences	21	19
Home cooked	5	7
Ease of preparation	5	4
Price	5	4
Baby's age	5	1
Other eg size of packet, shelf-life	20	12
Base:	4,591*	4,733*

* Bases are the reweighted numbers

The third stage questionnaires went on to ask mothers if they avoided giving foods which contained particular ingredients, and if so, why. When the baby was aged between 9–10 months 61% of mothers said that they did avoid particular ingredients and Table 6.11 shows which ingredients these were. When mothers said that they took sugar, salt or additives into account when deciding what food to give their baby it appears that they meant that they cut down on these things as these ingredients were the most commonly avoided.

Table 6.11 Ingredients avoided by mothers who gave solid food at nine months (1985 Great Britain)

Ingredients avoided	Percentage avoiding each ingredient
Sugar	55
Salt	35
Additives	31
Colourings	21
Preservatives	11
Fat	10
Flavourings	5
Other additives	2
Specific foodstuffs	30
Other	1
Base:	3,055*

Percentages do not add up to 100 as some mothers avoided more than one ingredient
* Base is the reweighted number

The majority of the reasons given for avoiding particular ingredients were rather general, 59% of mothers who avoided certain ingredients said it was because they thought them not beneficial, and 30% said they thought them harmful. Of the more specific reasons given, the most common was that it was 'bad for the teeth', 22% gave this as a reason presumably for avoiding sugar. Thus it appears that about a third of all mothers are deliberately avoiding sugar as they feel it is not good for the baby particularly the teeth. *Present day practice in infant feeding: third report*[5] sees this as a desirable feeding practice as it states that 'when solids are introduced, the regulation of sugar consumption is desirable so as to reduce the risk of dental caries and the possibility of obesity.'

6.5 Additional drinks

At all stages of the survey mothers were asked whether or not they gave their baby any additional drinks apart from milk. Table 6.12 shows that when the babies were about six weeks old 86% of them were receiving additional drinks, this was significantly lower than the 1980 figure of 88%. However it was only among babies that were being breast fed that this decrease occurred, 76% received additional drinks in 1980 compared with 68% in 1985. Among babies who were bottle fed there was no significant change, the respective figures were 95% and 94%. The 1980 survey found that bottle fed babies were more likely than breast fed babies to have been given additional drinks. This was still the case in 1985 and the difference between the two groups had increased; 94% of bottle fed babies compared with 68% of breast fed babies were receiving additional drinks.

Table 6.12 Additional drinks given to babies at about six weeks by feeding method (1980 and 1985 Great Britain)

	Breast fed		Bottle fed		All babies	
	1980	1985	1980	1985	1980	1985
	%	%	%	%	%	%
Drinks given	76	68	95	94	88	86
No drinks given	24	32	5	6	12	14
	100	100	100	100	100	100
Base:	1,520	1,719	2,704	3,504	4,224	5,223

By the time the babies were about four months old the proportion receiving additional drinks had risen to 91%. Bottle fed babies were still more likely than breast fed babies to have been given additional drinks; 94% compared with 82%. By the time they were nine months old virtually all babies, breast and bottle fed alike, were being given drinks in addition to milk (98%).

At each stage of the 1985 survey mothers were asked what types of drinks they gave their baby and their answers are shown in Table 6.13. At six weeks the majority of mothers who were giving drinks were giving their baby plain water, 52%, but a considerable number of mothers were giving sweetened baby drinks, for example 34% were giving special baby drinks sweetened with sugar or glucose. A quarter of mothers were giving a fennel drink, this was flavoured with herbs and contained sugar. Very few mothers were giving adult drinks at this age.

By the time the babies were four months old sweetened baby drinks and plain water were equally popular as additional drinks, 46% of mothers were giving each of these. Again a quarter of mothers were giving a fennel drink. When the babies were nine months old plain

Table 6.13 Types of non-milk drinks given at about six weeks (stage 1), four months (stage 2) and nine months (stage 3) (1985 Great Britain)

Type of drink given	Baby aged:		
	6 weeks	4 months	9 months
	Percentage giving each drink		
Plain water	52	46	47
Water with sugar/honey added	14	10	5
Baby drink with sugar/glucose	34	46	36
Baby drink with artificial sweetner	0	0	–
Baby drink unsweetened	7	14	14
Baby drink unspecified	5	13	19
Fennel drink	25	25	10
Adult drink with sugar/glucose	1	1	8
Adult drink with artificial sweetner	0	0	0
Adult drink unsweetened	2	5	19
Adult drink unspecified	1	8	30
Other drink	0	1	0
Base:	4,374	4,673*	5,096*

* Bases are the reweighted numbers

water and special baby drinks were still popular but a lot more mothers were giving adult drinks at this age; 19% said they were giving an unsweetened adult drink and 30% said they were giving some sort of adult drink, although they did not specify whether it was sweetened or not.

At six weeks and again at four months mothers who gave additional drinks were asked what their main reasons for doing so were. At both these ages the most common reason given was because the mother thought that the baby was thirsty, 77% gave this as a reason at six weeks and 81% at four months (Table 6.14). Most of the other reasons given were either to help the baby's digestion or to give it extra vitamins.

Table 6.14 Reasons for giving additional drinks at about six weeks (stage 1) and at about four months (stage 2) (1985 Great Britain)

Reasons for giving additional drinks	Baby aged:	
	6 weeks	4 months
	Percentage giving reason	
Because baby is thirsty	77	81
To give baby extra vitamins	13	20
To help baby's digestion	24	23
Other reason	4	9
Base:	4,419	4,615*

* Base is the reweighted number

6.6 Supplementary vitamins

Healthy infants born near term who are either breast fed or fed infant formula are unlikely to become vitamin deficient. However, it is important for older infants who are receiving milk that is unmodified for babies to receive supplements of vitamins. In order to safeguard all infants *Present day practice in infant feeding: third report*[5] recommends that vitamin supplements should be given to children aged from six months up to at least two years and preferably five years, and recognises and supports the fact that many professionals advise giving vitamin drops from the age of one month.

At the time of the survey children's vitamin drops (containing vitamins A, C and D) were available from child health clinics under the Welfare Food Scheme. Pregnant women and families with a child under five who were on supplementary benefit, or family income supplement, or whose income was low were entitled to these vitamins free of charge.

At all stages of the survey mothers were asked if they were giving their baby supplementary vitamins. When the babies were about six weeks old 27% of mothers were giving vitamin drops. This proportion had risen to 35% at four months and to 42% at nine months. At all three stages the vast majority of mothers who gave vitamin drops were using children's vitamin drops obtained at a child health clinic. Table 6.15 shows that mothers were most likely to buy the vitamins themselves at the clinic, although substantial minorities obtained them free of charge (or said they were on prescription). Only 4–5% of mothers who gave vitamin drops were buying other brands themselves.

Table 6.15 Type of vitamin drops given at about six weeks (stage 1), four months (stage 2), and nine months (stage 3) by mothers who gave them (1985 Great Britain)

Type of vitamins	Baby aged:		
	6 weeks	4 months	9 months
	%	%	%
Children's vitamin drops:	92	93	93
bought at clinic	49	50	64
free/prescribed at clinic	38	39	26
obtained elsewhere	5	4	3
Other brands:	8	7	7
bought	4	4	5
prescribed	4	3	2
Total	100	100	100
Base:	1,351	1,820*	2,200*

* Bases are the reweighted numbers

There were too few babies receiving liquid cow's milk at six weeks for this group to be analysed separately, so Table 6.16 compares the vitamin supplements received by breast fed and formula fed babies at about six weeks. Since 1980 there has been a considerable fall in the proportion of babies receiving vitamins at six weeks; only 27% did so in 1985 compared with 35% in 1980. This fall occurred among both breast fed and

Table 6.16 Supplementary vitamins given to babies of about six weeks by method of feeding (1980 and 1985 Great Britain)

	Breast fed		Bottle fed		All babies	
	1980	1985	1980	1985	1980	1985
	%	%	%	%	%	%
Received vitamins	47	34	29	23	35	27
Did not receive vitamins	53	66	71	77	65	73
	100	100	100	100	100	100
Base:	1,520	1,720	2,704	3,503	4,224	5,223

bottle fed babies. In 1985 breast fed babies were still more likely than bottle fed babies to have received vitamins as had been the case in 1980, 34% compared with 23%.

By the age of four months a similar pattern to that at six weeks was observed in that all babies, regardless of feeding method, were considerably less likely to be receiving vitamins than in 1980 (Table 6.17). Overall 35% of babies aged four months were being given vitamins in 1985 compared with 47% in 1980. By this age there were sufficient babies receiving liquid cow's milk for this group to be analysed separately and Table 6.17 shows that in 1985 less than half of them (44%) were being given vitamin supplements. Among breast fed babies the proportion receiving vitamins at this age was 45%, virtually the same as among those receiving liquid cow's milk, but among those receiving infant formula only 32% were being given vitamins.

The 1980 survey did not collect information on whether vitamins were being given when the baby was nine months old but in 1985 among both breast fed babies and those receiving liquid cow's milk the proportions receiving vitamins was virtually the same at nine months as it had been at four months, 45% among each group. However, among those receiving infant formula the proportion had increased from 32% at four months to 37% at nine months (Table 6.18).

6.7 Problems with feeding when the baby was aged four months and nine months

When the babies were about four months old 22% of mothers said that they had experienced some problems feeding their baby. Bottle feeding mothers were slightly more likely than breast feeding mothers to say that they had experienced problems, 23% compared with 20%.

Table 6.17 Supplementary vitamins given to babies of about four months by method of feeding (1980 and 1985 Great Britain)

	Breast fed		Bottle fed:				All babies†	
			liquid cows milk		infant formula			
	1980	1985	1980	1985	1980	1985	1980	1985
	%	%	%	%	%	%	%	%
Received vitamins	66	45	57	44	39	32	47	35
Did not receive vitamins	34	55	43	56	61	68	53	65
	100	100	100	100	100	100	100	100
Base:	1,021*	1,187*	178*	239*	2,969*	3,701*	4,224*	5,223*

† Includes some babies who received only non-human milk for which the type was not known
* Bases are the reweighted numbers

Table 6.18 Supplementary vitamins given to babies of about nine months by method of feeding (1985 Great Britain)

	Breast fed	Bottle fed:		All babies†
		liquid cows milk	infant formula	
	%	%	%	%
Received vitamins	45	45	37	42
Did not receive vitamins	55	55	63	58
	100	100	100	100
Base:	462*	3,072*	1,508*	5,223*

† Includes some babies who received only non-human milk for which the type was not known
* Bases are the reweighted numbers

Table 6.19 Feeding problems experienced by mothers when babies were about four months old (stage 2) and nine months old (stage 3) (1985 Great Britain)

Type of problem	Baby aged:					
	Four months			Nine months		
	Breast fed	Bottle fed	All babies	Breast fed	Bottle fed	All babies
	Percentage having problem					
Baby hungry	25	18	19	1	3	3
Baby ill	9	17	15	9	14	13
Baby did not like milk	17	15	15	14	6	7
Baby vomiting	4	20	17	1	7	6
Baby got too much/ too little wind	5	4	4	3	0	0
Baby constipated	5	7	7	1	3	3
Sore/cracked nipples	8	2	3	2	0	0
Baby could not latch on	1	0	0	–	–	–
Baby would not take solids	12	10	11	16	9	10
Baby would only take certain solids	6	10	9	17	31	29
Baby not hungry	..	..	..	2	8	7
Baby teething	..	..	..	3	7	7
Baby allergic to milk	..	..	..	2	3	3
Baby allergic to other foods	..	..	..	2	3	3
Other	27	10	14	36	18	21
Base:	224*	823*	1,046*	110*	657*	767*

Percentages do not add up to 100 as some mothers experienced more than one type of feeding problem
* Bases are the reweighted numbers

Table 6.19 shows the problems that these mothers had. Many of the problems mentioned were similar to those experienced when the baby was younger, the most common was the baby being hungry, 19% of those who had problems mentioned this. Problems with giving solid food began to feature at this age, 11% of mothers who had problems said that the baby would not take solid food and 9% said it would only take certain solids. Most mothers who had problems received help or advice from someone else (84%) and in most cases the adviser was the health visitor; 57% were advised by her.

By the time the babies were nine months old only 15% of mothers reported having problems feeding their baby, breast feeders being more likely to have done so than bottle feeders, 24% compared with 14%. Table 6.19 shows the problems experienced at this age, the most common problems mentioned were to do with giving solid food. Twenty nine per cent said their baby would only take certain solids and 10% said their baby wouldn't take solid food. Again the majority of mothers received help with these problems (66%), usually from the health visitor.

6.8 Problems with feeding and changing the baby in public places

On the stage 2 questionnaire, when the babies were about four months old, mothers were asked whether they had ever had any problems finding somewhere to feed or change their baby when out in public places. Overall about a third of mothers said that they had problems finding somewhere to feed their baby and almost half of them said that they had problems finding somewhere to change their baby when out in public places (Table 6.20). In addition a considerable number of mothers said that they only went out in between feeds (34%) or that they never tried to change the baby when out in public places (28%). Even among breast feeding mothers, problems with finding somewhere to change the baby were mentioned more often than problems with finding somewhere to feed it.

Not surprisingly breast feeding mothers were more likely than those who were bottle feeding to have experienced problems finding somewhere to feed their baby, 50% compared with 27%.

Table 6.20 Whether mothers ever had any problems finding somewhere to feed or change their babies in public places (1985 Great Britain)

| | Whether had problems finding somewhere to: | | | | | |
| | Feed baby | | | Change baby | | |
	Breast feeders	Bottle feeders	All mothers	Breast feeders	Bottle feeders	All mothers
	%	%	%	%	%	%
Had problems	50	27	32	53	47	48
Did not have problems	22	38	34	20	25	22
Do not feed/change in public places	28	35	34	27	28	28
	100	100	100	100	100	100
Base:	*1,191**	*4,032**	*5,233**	*1,191**	*4,032**	*5,233**

* Bases are the reweighted numbers

Table 6.21 Places that mothers thought should provide facilities for feeding and changing babies (1985 Great Britain)

| | Places that mothers thought should provide: | | | | | |
| | Facilities for feeding babies | | | Facilities for changing babies | | |
	Breast feeders	Bottle feeders	All mothers	Breast feeders	Bottle feeders	All mothers
	Percentage mentioning each place					
Shops/shopping centres	95	85	87	91	77	81
Restaurants	58	52	53	54	42	45
Public toilets	32	20	23	61	57	58
Stations and airports	8	2	4	7	2	3
Places of entertainment, eg parks, museums	6	2	3	5	1	2
Other public places	7	4	5	5	4	4
Base:	*1,191**	*4,032**	*5,233**	*1,191**	*4,032**	*5,233**

* Bases are the reweighted numbers

Mothers were asked where they thought it was important to have facilities for feeding and for changing babies and their replies are shown in Table 6.21. The first three places shown in the table, shops and shopping centres, restaurants and public toilets were asked about specifically so it is not surprising that more mothers thought that these places should provide facilities than the other places shown in the table. It seems that most mothers would welcome more facilities both for feeding and for changing babies, shops and shopping centres were the places mentioned most often. *Present day practice in infant feeding: third report*[5] urges social, community, educational, commercial and other concerns to take a positive approach to enable mothers to feed and change their babies when and where this becomes necessary.

6.9 Care for the baby while the mother is working

As Chapter 2 showed, only 5% of mothers were work-ing when their baby was about six weeks old. At four months and at nine months the proportions of mothers who were working were still relatively low; 14% at four months and 20% at nine months. At both these ages mothers who were working were asked who usually looked after their baby while they were at work. Their answers are shown in Table 6.22. Relatives were the most likely people to look after the baby at four months, 29% of mothers left their baby in the care of their mother or mother-in-law and 26% in the care of their husband or partner. Nineteen per cent had a childminder to look after the baby and only 1% left it in a nursery or creche. Mothers who were breast feeding were more likely than those who were bottle feeding to leave their baby with a childminder or look after it themselves while they were at work rather than have relatives look after it. This probably reflects the fact that breast feeding mothers were more likely to be in the higher social classes and would therefore be more

Table 6.22 Who usually looks after the baby while the mother is working (1985 Great Britain)

| Person who looked after the baby | Baby aged: | | | | | |
| | Four months | | | Nine months | | |
	Breast feeders	Bottle feeders	All mothers	Breast feeders	Bottle feeders	All mothers
	%	%	%	%	%	%
Mother herself: homeworker	}17	}9	}11	21	7	8
out to work				3	2	2
Mother's husband/partner	19	28	26	15	32	31
Mother's mother/ mother-in-law	19	33	29	17	28	27
Child minder	23	18	19	31	20	21
Nursery/creche	1	1	1	–	2	2
Other	21	11	14	13	9	9
Base:	*175**	*558**	*733**	*81**	*980**	*1,061**

* Bases are the reweighted numbers

likely to be able to afford to pay for a childminder, or to have the sort of jobs whereby they could look after the baby themselves, for example, working from home. Of those who had their baby looked after by someone other than themselves or their husband or partner 67% paid for child care, breast feeding mothers being more likely to do so than bottle feeding mothers, 81% compared with 63%.

When the baby was nine months old the pattern of child care adopted by working mothers was much the same as it had been at four months; breast feeding mothers were more likely to have a childminder or to look after the baby themselves and bottle feeders were more likely to have relatives looking after the baby. Table 6.22 shows that when the babies were nine months old 21% of breast feeders compared with 7% of bottle feeders looked after their baby themselves while working from home. Again breast feeding mothers were more likely than those who were bottle feeding to pay for child care, 73% compared with 66%. Working mothers who were still breast feeding when the baby was about nine months old were asked how they usually fed their baby while they were at work. The majority, 57% said that the baby had other milk while they were at work, 7% said they were able to feed the baby while at work and the rest had some other arrangement.

References

1   Jean Martin. *Infant feeding 1975: attitudes and practice in England and Wales*, HMSO (1978).

2   Jean Martin and Janet Monk. *Infant feeding 1980*, HMSO (1982).

3   *Present day practice in infant feeding*. Report on Health and Social Subjects 9, DHSS (1974).

4   *Present day practice in infant feeding 1980*. Report on Health and Social Subjects 20, DHSS (1980).

5   *Present day practice in infant feeding: third report*. Report on Health and Social Subjects 32, DHSS (1988).

6   World Health Organisation. *International code of marketing of breast-milk substitutes*. World Health Organisation (Geneva 1981).

Appendix I Composition of the 1985 sample compared with the 1980 sample and with the 1985 population estimates

Table I.1 Distribution of the population and the sample by birth order (1980 and 1985 Great Britain)

Birth order	Population*		Surveys	
	1980	1985	1980	1985
	%	%	%	%
First birth	43	40	44	46
Second birth	36	36	36	33
Third birth	14	16	13	14
Fourth birth	}7	}8	5}7	5}7
Fifth or later birth			2}	2}
	100	100	100	100
Base:	*601,600*	*584,500*	*4,224*	*5,223*

* *Figures based on legitimate live births only*

Table I.2 Distribution of the sample by mother's main occupation (1980 and 1985 Great Britain)

Main occupation	1980	1985
	%	%
Professional	1	1
Teaching	6	5
Nursing, medical or social	8	7
Other managerial or intermediate non-manual	5	6
Clerical	34	28
Shop assistant or related sales	7	9
Total non-manual	**61**	**55**
Skilled manual	9	6
Semi-skilled factory work	12	12
Semi-skilled domestic work	3	5
Other semi-skilled	2	2
Unskilled	1	1
Total manual	**27**	**26**
Not classified	12	18
	100	100
Base:	*4,224*	*5,223*

Table I.3 Distribution of the sample by age at which mother finished full-time education, for first and later births (1980 and 1985 Great Britain)

Mother's age at finishing full-time education	First births		Later births		All babies	
	1980	1985	1980	1985	1980	1985
	%	%	%	%	%	%
16 or under	59	56	66	63	63	60
17 or 18	25	30	19	23	21	26
Over 18	16	14	15	14	16	14
	100	100	100	100	100	100
Base:	*1,831*	*2,336*	*2,337*	*2,845*	*4,224*	*5,223*

Table I.4 Distribution of social class by age at which mother finished full-time education (1980 and 1985 Great Britain)

Social class		Mother's age at finishing full-time education							
		16 or under		17 or 18		Over 18		All ages	
		1980	1985	1980	1985	1980	1985	1980	1985
		%	%	%	%	%	%	%	%
I	Professional	3	2	8	7	29	21	8	6
II	Managerial and technical	12	12	23	24	38	46	18	20
IIINM	Clerical and minor supervisory	8	8	11	11	9	8	8	8
Total non-manual		**22**	**21**	**42**	**42**	**76**	**75**	**34**	**34**
IIIM	Skilled manual	49	37	40	31	16	13	42	32
IV	Semi-skilled manual	16	17	10	13	3	6	13	14
V	Unskilled manual	4	6	2	4	–	–	3	5
Total manual		**69**	**60**	**52**	**48**	**19**	**19**	**58**	**51**
Unclassified		.. }9	5 }19	.. }6	2 }10	.. }5	4 }6	.. }8	4 }15
No partner		..	14	..	8	..	3	..	11
		100	100	100	100	100	100	100	100
Base:		2,632	3,110	892	1,346	657	725	4,224	5,223

Table I.5 Distribution of the population and the sample by mother's age (1980 and 1985 Great Britain)

Mother's age	Population*		Surveys	
	1980	1985	1980	1985
	%	%	%	%
Under 20	9	9	8	8
20–24	31	30	31	30
25–29	34	35	36	35
30 or over	26	27	25	27
	100	100	100	100
Base:	725,000	723,100	4,224	5,223

* *Figures based on all live births*

Table I.6 Distribution of the sample by mother's age, for first and later births (1980 and 1985 Great Britain)

Mother's age	First births		Later births		All babies	
	1980	1985	1980	1985	1980	1985
	%	%	%	%	%	%
Under 20	15	16	2	2	8	8
20–24	40	38	24	23	31	30
25–29	33	31	38	38	36	35
30 or over	12	14	36	38	25	27
	100	100	100	100	100	100
Base:	1,831	2,343	2,377	2,864	4,224	5,223

Table I.7 Age of mothers of first babies by social class (1980 and 1985 Great Britain)

Mother's age	Social class									
	I		II		IIINM		IIIM		IV and V	
	1980	1985	1980	1985	1980	1985	1980	1985	1980	1985
	%	%	%	%	%	%	%	%	%	%
Under 20	–	2	3	3	4	4	15	10	23	22
20–24	15	16	27	25	33	33	50	46	48	47
25–29	52	49	51	42	49	44	27	34	21	24
30 or over	33	32	19	30	14	19	8	9	8	8
	100	100	100	100	100	100	100	100	100	100
Base:	138	136	311	444	179	213	742	703	266	386

Table I.8 Age of mothers of first babies by age at finishing full-time education (1980 and 1985 Great Britain)

Mother's age	Mother's age at finishing full-time education					
	16 or under		17 or 18		Over 18	
	1980	1985	1980	1985	1980	1985
	%	%	%	%	%	%
Under 20	21	23	11	10	–	0
20–24	44	42	44	42	21	15
25–29	26	25	35	35	56	47
30 or over	9	9	10	13	23	37
	100	100	100	100	100	100
Base:	*1,067*	*1,309*	*453*	*697*	*298*	*328*

Table I.9 Distribution of the sample by region (1980 and 1985 Great Britain)

Region	1980	1985
	%	%
London and South East	30	32
South West and Wales	11	13
Midlands and East Anglia	19	18
North	30	26
Scotland	11	11
	100	100
Base:	*4,224*	*5,223*

Table I.10 Distribution of birth order by region (1980 and 1985 Great Britain)

Birth order	Region									
	London and South East		South West and Wales		Midlands and East Anglia		North		Scotland	
	1980	1985	1980	1985	1980	1985	1980	1985	1980	1985
	%	%	%	%	%	%	%	%	%	%
First birth	45	45	41	45	43	44	44	46	42	46
Second and subsequent birth	55	55	59	55	57	56	56	54	58	54
	100	100	100	100	100	100	100	100	100	100
Base:	*1,284*	*1,675*	*483*	*657*	*808*	*960*	*1,179*	*1,378*	*1,718*	*1,895*

Table I.11 Distribution of social class by region (1980 and 1985 Great Britain)

Social class	Region									
	London and South East		South West and Wales		Midlands and East Anglia		North		Scotland	
	1980	1985	1980	1985	1980	1985	1980	1985	1980	1985
	%	%	%	%	%	%	%	%	%	%
I	11	8	9	6	5	4	6	4	8	6
II	22	25	15	19	19	18	16	16	16	16
IIINM	9	9	9	9	8	6	8	9	7	9
Total non-manual	**42**	**42**	**33**	**34**	**32**	**28**	**30**	**29**	**31**	**32**
IIIM	38	30	43	32	44	38	44	30	41	33
IV	9	10	16	15	13	17	14	17	15	13
V	2	4	2	5	2	3	4	6	5	7
Total manual	**49**	**43**	**61**	**52**	**59**	**58**	**62**	**53**	**61**	**53**
Unclassified	‥ ⎱9	4 ⎱14	‥ ⎱6	3 ⎱14	‥ ⎱9	4 ⎱15	‥ ⎱8	4 ⎱18	‥ ⎱8	3 ⎱15
No husband	‥ ⎰	10 ⎰	‥ ⎰	10 ⎰	‥ ⎰	10 ⎰	‥ ⎰	13 ⎰	‥ ⎰	12 ⎰
	100	100	100	100	100	100	100	100	100	100
Base:	*1,284*	*1,675*	*483*	*657*	*808*	*960*	*1,179*	*1,378*	*1,718*	*1,895*

Table I.12 Distribution of mother's age at finishing full-time education by region (1980 and 1985 Great Britain)

Mother's age at finishing full-time education	Region									
	London and South East		South West and Wales		Midlands and East Anglia		North		Scotland	
	1980	1985	1980	1985	1980	1985	1980	1985	1980	1985
	%	%	%	%	%	%	%	%	%	%
16 or under	55	52	61	55	67	64	69	69	65	63
17 or 18	25	29	25	31	19	26	18	21	19	23
Over 18	20	19	14	14	14	10	13	11	16	14
	100	100	100	100	100	100	100	100	100	100
Base:	*1,284*	*1,662*	*483*	*654*	*808*	*950*	*1,179*	*1,364*	*1,718*	*1,895*

Appendix II Sampling errors

Since the design of the sample was two-stage and stratified it was necessary to calculate sampling errors using a formula which took this into account. Table II.1 shows estimates of the sampling errors relating to the incidence of breast feeding for each of the main sub-groups included in the analysis.

Table II.1 Sampling errors for the incidence of breast feeding (1985 Great Britain)

		Incidence	Sampling error
Total sample		64%	1.20%
Social class	I	87%	2.04%
	II	81%	1.40%
	IIINM	76%	2.44%
	IIIM	61%	1.58%
	IV & V	54%	2.07%
Region	London and South East	74%	1.59%
	South West and Wales	68%	3.75%
	Midlands and East Anglia	62%	2.26%
	North	56%	2.49%
	Scotland	48%	..
Age at which mother finished full-time education	16 or under	53%	1.42%
	17 or 18	75%	1.18%
	Over 18	89%	1.22%
Birth order	First birth	69%	1.45%
	Later birth	59%	1.33%

Appendix III Survey documents

Five versions of the questionnaire were used, of which three are included here:

(a) the original questionnaire sent to all mothers at six weeks (stage 1),

(b) the questionnaire sent at four months to mothers who had been breast feeding at the time of completing the first questionnaire (stage 2),

(c) the questionnaire sent at nine months to mothers who had been breast feeding at the time of completing the second questionnaire (stage 3).

Those questionnaires not included here differed from the others only in questions omitted.

Twelve different covering letters were used according to the stage of the survey, whether it was the initial approach or a reminder, and depending on whether the baby was born in England and Wales or Scotland. Three of the letters are included here:

(a) the initial letter at six weeks

(b) the initial letter at four months

(c) the initial letter at nine months

(a) Stage 1 documents: initial letter and questionnaire

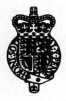

Office of Population Censuses and Surveys
Social Survey Division
St Catherines House   10 Kingsway   London   WC2B 6JP
Telephone 01-242 0262   ext   2256

Your reference

Our reference   S 1233/E1/1

Date   Sept/Oct   1985

Dear Madam

SURVEY OF INFANT FEEDING

I am writing to ask for your help in an enquiry into Infant Feeding that is being carried out for the Department of Health and Social Security, since I understand that you have recently had a baby. A survey on the same subject was carried out in 1980 and we want to find out how practices have changed since then.

We would like to hear from mothers of young babies about how they feed their babies. Since we cannot contact all mothers we have selected names at random from the register of births and your name has been included by chance in this selection.

I realise how busy you are at the moment with a new baby but I would be very grateful if you could spare time to fill in the enclosed questionnaire and return it in the envelope provided.

If, for any reason, your baby is no longer with you please tick the box on the front page of the questionnaire and return it to us so that we do not trouble you further.

As in all our surveys we rely on people's voluntary co-operation. The information that you give is treated in strict confidence by OPCS. It is not released to any other Government department in any way in which it can be associated with your name and address. No information about your household is ever passed to members of the public or press. In published reports the identity of an individual is never revealed: the results of the survey are shown as statistics only.

Thank you in advance for your help.

Yours faithfully

Lizanne Dowds

Lizanne Dowds
Research Officer

61

S1233/1   01 = 1/2
SERNO = 3-6
SAMPNO = 7-14

SURVEY OF INFANT FEEDING

1. Most questions on the following pages can be answered simply by putting a tick in the box next to the answer that applies to you.

Example:

Yes ✓ 1

No ☐ 2

Sometimes you are asked to write in a number or the answer in your own words. Please enter numbers as figures rather than words.

2. Usually after answering each question you go on to the next one unless a box you have ticked has an arrow next to it with an instruction to go to another question

Example:

Yes ✓ 1 → Q5

No ☐ 2

By following the arrows carefully you will miss out some questions which do not apply to you, so the amount you have to fill in will make the questionnaire shorter than it looks.

3. If you cannot remember, do not know, or are unable to answer a particular question please write that in.

4. If, rather than a single baby, you have twins or triplets, please answer the questions in relation to the one who was born first.

5. When you have finished please post the questionnaire to us as soon as possible in the reply-paid envelope provided, even if you were not able to answer all of it.

The names and addresses of people who co-operate in surveys are held in strict confidence by OPCS and never passed to any other Government Department, or to members of the public or press.

We shall be very grateful for your help.

If for any reason your baby is not with you at the moment please tick the box below and return the questionnaire to us so we do not trouble you further.

My baby is no longer with me ☐

---

6. (a) How old was your baby when you last breast fed him/her?

PLEASE ENTER NUMBERS IN BOTH BOXES

weeks [ ] and [ ] days

23-25

(b) What were your reasons for stopping breast feeding?
(Please give all your reasons and explain)

MC=5

26-35

7. Which kind of milk do you give your baby at the moment?

36/37

Cow and Gate Premium	01
Cow and Gate Plus	02
Cow and Gate Formula S	03
Osterfeed baby milk	04
Ostermilk complete formula	05
Ostermilk Two	06
SMA Gold Cap	07
SMA White Cap	08
Wysoy	09
Milupa Milumil	10
Milupa Aptamil	11
Another kind of milk (please tick and write in the name)	12

PLEASE TICK ONE BOX ONLY

If you use liquid cow's milk please say if it is ordinary (whole) milk, semi-skimmed or skimmed.

3

First of all, we would like to ask some general questions before finding out how you feed your baby at present.

1. How old is your baby?

PLEASE ENTER NUMBERS IN BOTH BOXES

weeks [ ] and [ ] days

15-17

2. Is this your first baby?

Yes [1]
No [2]

18

3. Is he/she one of twins or triplets?

No, neither [1]
Yes, twin [2]
Yes, triplet [3]

19

4. At the moment is your baby .....

breast fed [1] →(a)
bottle fed [2] →Q5
or both? [3] →Q7

20

(a) Do you give him/her milk in a bottle at present (apart from expressed breast milk)?

Yes (even if only occasionally) [1] →Q7
No [2] →Q11

21

5. Did you ever put your baby to the breast?

Yes (even if it was once only) [1] →Q6
No, never [2] →Q7

22

2

8. Have you always used the milk mentioned at question 7 or have you changed milks at all (apart from changing from breast milk)?

Have always used the same milk [1] → Q11

Have used other milks [2] → Q9

Please do not write in this column

38

9. Please list in order all the other milks you have used. Include any milks used in hospital, but exclude breast milk.

Please give full brand name, as on the list at question 7.

For each milk you have used please tick boxes to show the reasons you stopped using it, or write in the reason.

DO NOT INCLUDE THE MILK YOU USE AT PRESENT

FIRST TYPE OF MILK

Reason for stopping using this milk

Baby not satisfied/still hungry [1] 39/40

Baby kept being sick [2] MC=3

Baby was constipated [3] 41-43

Baby was allergic to this milk [4]

Other reason (please write in) [5]

SECOND TYPE OF MILK

Baby not satisfied/still hungry [1] 44/45

Baby kept being sick [2] MC=3

Baby was constipated [3] 46-48

Baby was allergic to this milk [4]

Other reason (please write in) [5]

THIRD TYPE OF MILK

Baby not satisfied/still hungry [1] 49/50

Baby kept being sick [2] MC=3

Baby was constipated [3] 51-53

Baby was allergic to this milk [4]

Other reason (please write in) [5]

FOURTH TYPE OF MILK

Baby not satisfied/still hungry [1] 54/55

Baby kept being sick [2] MC=3

Baby was constipated [3] 56-58

Baby was allergic to this milk [4]

Other reason (please write in) [5]

4

10. Did any of these people advise you to change milks, at any time?

No-one advised me [1] MC=4

Health Visitor [2] 59-62

Midwife/nurse [3]

Doctor [4]

Friend or relative [5]

Someone else (please tick and write in) [6]

11. Do you get milk tokens?

Yes - for the baby [1] MC=3

Yes - for myself [2] 63-65

Yes - for older child [3]

Have applied for tokens [4]

No - I don't get tokens [5]

12. Has your baby ever had any foods such as cereal, rusk or any other kind of solid food?

Yes [1] → (a) - (b)   66

No [2] → Q15

(a) How old was your baby when he/she first had any food apart from milk?   PLEASE ENTER A NUMBER IN THE BOX

[ ] weeks old   67/68

(b) What was the first food he/she had, apart from milk?

PLEASE DESCRIBE FULLY

TYPE OF FOOD _____

BRAND (or say if home made) _____

69/70

END 01

5

16. Do you give your baby drinks mainly....

because he/she is thirsty [1]

to give him/her extra vitamins [2]

to help his/her colic/wind [3]

to help his/her constipation [4]

or for some other reason (please tick and write in) [5]

17. Do you give your baby any extra vitamins (apart from vitamin drinks mentioned at question 15)?

Yes [1] → (a) - (b)

No [2] → Q18

33

(a) Do you use Children's Vitamin Drops from the clinic or another brand?

Children's Vitamin Drops [1]

Other brand (please tick and write in full name) [2]

34

(b) How do you get the vitamins?

Buy the vitamins myself [1]

Get vitamins free at the clinic [2]

Get vitamins on prescription [3]

Other (please tick and describe) [4]

35

18. Do you feed your baby on demand or do you generally keep to set feeding times?

On demand [1]

Generally keep to set times [2]

It depends on the circumstances [3]

36

7

---

13. At present, are you regularly giving your baby cereal, rusks or any other solid food?

Yes [1] → Q14

No [2] → Q15

8

14. Thinking back to yesterday, can you list all the cereal, rusks or solid food that your baby ate. Please describe each fully, giving the brand name and the stage (1 or 2) if relevant.

Didn't have solids yesterday [1] → Q15

TYPE OF FOOD (AND STAGE)	BRAND (OR HOME MADE)

MC=6

9-20

15. Apart from milk, do you give your baby water or anything else to drink?

Yes [1] → (a)

No [2] → Q1

21

(a) Please tick boxes or write in the drink your baby usually has. Please give the brand name, flavour and say if it is a special baby drink or not.

Plain water [1]

Water with sugar or honey added [2]

PLEASE TICK IF IT IS A BABY DRINK

22

BRAND NAME	FLAVOUR

MC=3

23-28

6

65

Now a few questions about when you were pregnant.

19. Thinking back to before you had your baby, how did you plan to feed him/her?

Bottle feed [1]
Breast feed [2] → (a)
Had not decided [3] → Q20

(a) Why did you think you would feed him/her by that method?
(Please explain all your reasons)

20. While you were pregnant did you have any antenatal checkups?

Yes [1]
No [2]

(a) When you went for your checkups did anyone ask how you planned to feed the baby?

Yes [1]
No [2]

(b) At the checkups did anyone discuss feeding the baby with you?

Yes [1]
No [2]

21. While you were pregnant with this baby did you go to any classes on parentcraft or to prepare you for having the baby?

Yes [1] → Q22
No [2] → Q24

8

Please do not write in this column

37

MC=5

38-47

48

49

50

51

22. (a) Who were the classes organised by?

A hospital [1]
A clinic [2]
Another organisation (Please tick and give name) [3]

(b) Did you attend any classes that included talks or discussions about feeding babies?

Yes [1] → Q23
No [2] → Q24

23. (a) Did the classes talk about advantages of breast feeding?

Yes [1]
No [2]

(b) Were you taught how to make up bottles of milk at the classes you attended?

Yes [1]
No [2]

24. (a) When you were pregnant were you given a copy of ......

The Pregnancy Book (Health Education Council) [1]
The Book of the Child (Scottish Health Education Group) [2]
Neither [3]

(b) Were you given any other free books or pamphlets which included information about feeding babies?

Yes [1]
No [2]

25. Did a midwife or health visitor see you at home in connection with your pregnancy before you had the baby?

Yes, midwife [1]
Yes, health visitor [2]
No, neither [3]

9

Please do not write in this column

MC=2
52/53

54

55

56

57

58

MC=2
59-60

30. How much did your baby weigh when he/she was born?

EITHER lbs [ ] and ozs [ ]

PLEASE ENTER NUMBERS IN THE BOXES

OR gms [ ]

11-14

31. (a) What time was your baby born?

PLEASE ENTER TIME IN APPROPRIATE BOX

am [ ] OR pm [ ]

15-18

19-22

(b) About how long after he/she was born did you first hold him/her?

immediately/within a few minutes [1]

within an hour [2]

more than 1 hour, up to 12 hours [3]

More than 12 hours later [4]

23

32. After the birth were you alright or was anything the matter with you?

Alright [1] → Q33

Something the matter [2] → (a)

24

(a) Did this problem affect your ability to feed your baby the way you wanted to?

Yes [1]

No [2]

25

33. Immediately after the birth did your baby have any problems which affected his/her feeding?

Yes [1] → (a)

No [2] → Q34

26

(a) What problems did he/she have?

MC=3

27-32

11

Please do not write in this column

26. When you were at school did you have any lessons on parentcraft or child development or anything like that?

Yes [1]

No [2]

61

27. Was your baby born at home or in hospital?

At home [1] → Q28

In hospital [2] → (a) - (b)

62

(a) How long after the baby was born did you stay in hospital?

PLEASE ENTER NUMBER IN ONE BOX ONLY

hours [ ] or days [ ]

63/64

(b) Was this .....

longer than you expected when you were pregnant [1]

shorter than you expected [2]

or about what you expected? [3]

65/66

67

28. Thinking now of the birth itself, what type of delivery did you have?

Normal [1]

Forceps [2]

Vacuum extraction [3]

Caesarean [4]

68

29. While you were in labour were you given any of these:

An epidural (spinal) injection [1]

PLEASE TICK ALL THAT APPLY

Another type of injection to lessen the pain (eg pethedine) [2]

Gas and oxygen to breathe [3]

A general anaesthetic (to make you unconscious) [4]

Something else (please tick and write in) [5]

Nothing at all [6]

MC=5

69-73

10

END 02

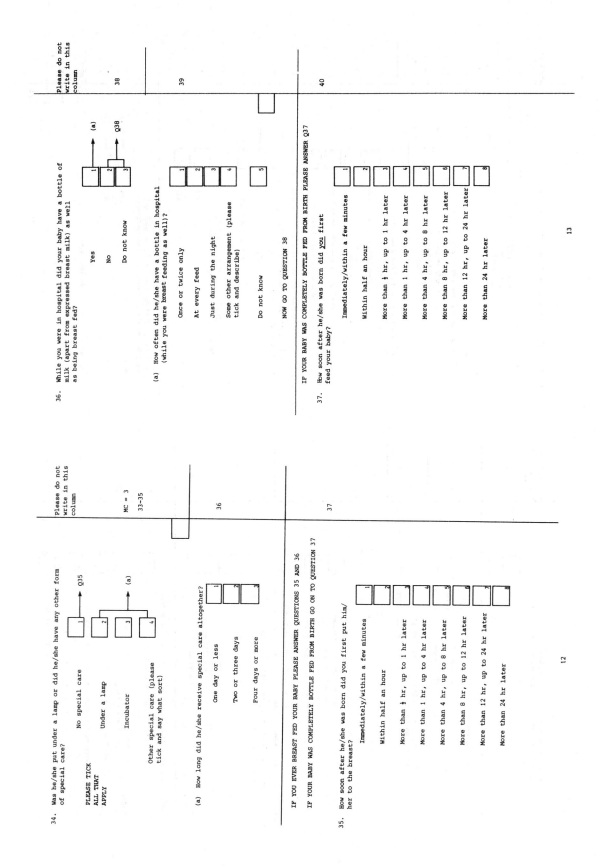

Page 12

34. Was he/she put under a lamp or did he/she have any other form of special care?

PLEASE TICK ALL THAT APPLY

No special care [1] → Q35

Under a lamp [2]

Incubator [3] → (a)

Other special care (please tick and say what sort) [4]

(a) How long did he/she receive special care altogether?

One day or less [1]

Two or three days [2]

Four days or more [3]

IF YOU EVER BREAST FED YOUR BABY PLEASE ANSWER QUESTIONS 35 AND 36

IF YOUR BABY WAS COMPLETELY BOTTLE FED FROM BIRTH GO ON TO QUESTION 37

35. How soon after he/she was born did you first put him/her to the breast?

Immediately/within a few minutes [1]

Within half an hour [2]

More than ½ hr, up to 1 hr later [3]

More than 1 hr, up to 4 hr later [4]

More than 4 hr, up to 8 hr later [5]

More than 8 hr, up to 12 hr later [6]

More than 12 hr, up to 24 hr later [7]

More than 24 hr later [8]

Please do not write in this column

MC = 3

33-35

36

37

12

Page 13

36. While you were in hospital did your baby have a bottle of milk (apart from expressed breast milk) as well as being breast fed?

Yes [1] → (a)

No [2] → Q38

Do not know [3]

(a) How often did he/she have a bottle in hospital (while you were breast feeding as well)?

Once or twice only [1]

At every feed [2]

Just during the night [3]

Some other arrangement (please tick and describe) [4]

Do not know [5]

NOW GO TO QUESTION 38

IF YOUR BABY WAS COMPLETELY BOTTLE FED FROM BIRTH PLEASE ANSWER Q37

37. How soon after he/she was born did you first feed your baby?

Immediately/within a few minutes [1]

Within half an hour [2]

More than ½ hr, up to 1 hr later [3]

More than 1 hr, up to 4 hr later [4]

More than 4 hr, up to 8 hr later [5]

More than 8 hr, up to 12 hr later [6]

More than 12 hr, up to 24 hr later [7]

More than 24 hr later [8]

Please do not write in this column

38

39

40

13

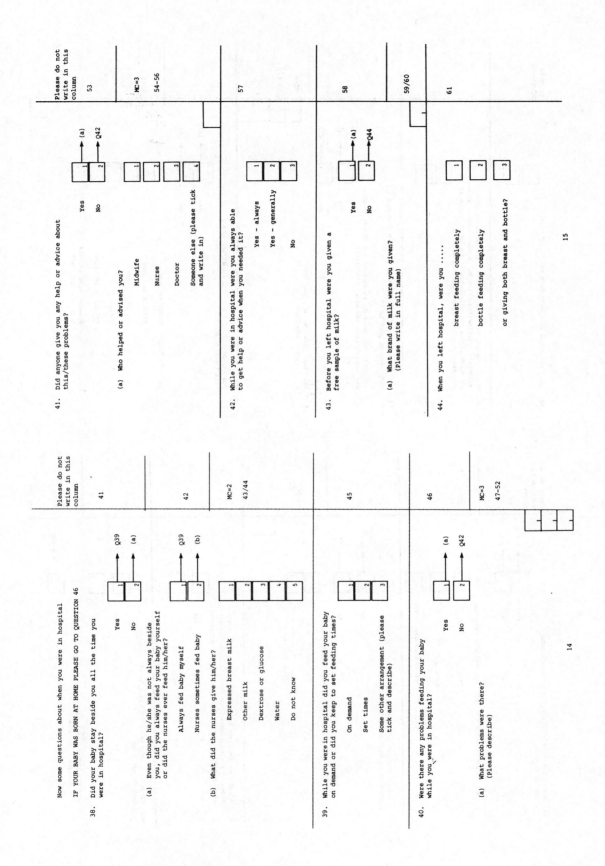

Now some questions about when you were in hospital

IF YOUR BABY WAS BORN AT HOME PLEASE GO TO QUESTION 46

38. Did your baby stay beside you all the time you were in hospital?

Yes [1] → Q39
No [2] → (a)

(a) Even though he/she was not always beside you, did you always feed your baby yourself or did the nurses ever feed him/her?

Always fed baby myself [1] → Q39
Nurses sometimes fed baby [2] → (b)

(b) What did the nurses give him/her?

Expressed breast milk [1]
Other milk [2]
Dextrose or glucose [3]
Water [4]
Do not know [5]

39. While you were in hospital did you feed your baby on demand or did you keep to set feeding times?

On demand [1]
Set times [2]
Some other arrangement (please tick and describe) [3]

40. Were there any problems feeding your baby while you were in hospital?

Yes [1] → (a)
No [2] → Q42

(a) What problems were there? (Please describe)

Please do not write in this column

41
42
MC=2 43/44
45
46
MC=3 47-52

14

41. Did anyone give you any help or advice about this/these problems?

Yes [1] → (a)
No [2] → Q42

(a) Who helped or advised you?

Midwife [1]
Nurse [2]
Doctor [3]
Someone else (please tick and write in) [4]

42. While you were in hospital were you always able to get help or advice when you needed it?

Yes - always [1]
Yes - generally [2]
No [3]

43. Before you left hospital were you given a free sample of milk?

Yes [1] → (a)
No [2] → Q44

(a) What brand of milk were you given? (Please write in full name)

44. When you left hospital, were you ......

breast feeding completely [1]
bottle feeding completely [2]
or giving both breast and bottle? [3]

Please do not write in this column

53
MC=3 54-56
57
58
59/60
61

15

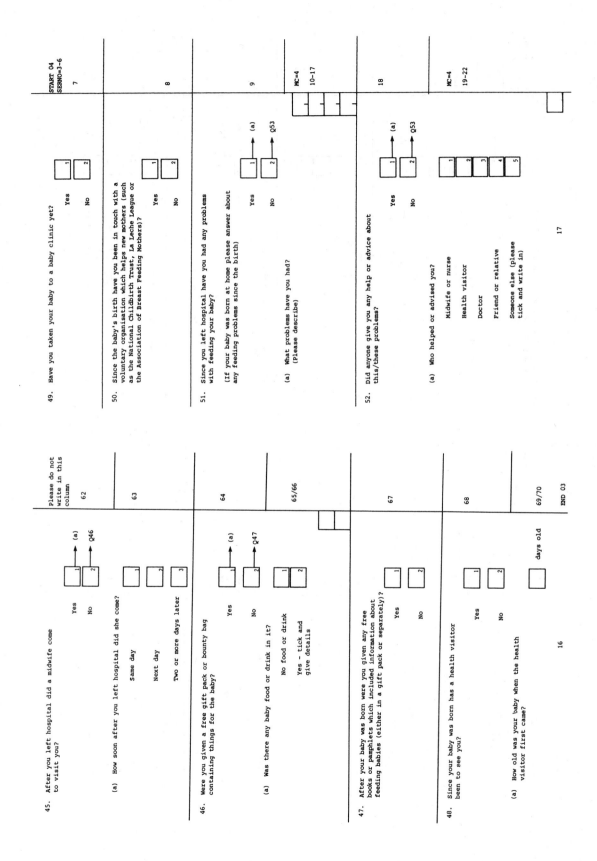

45. After you left hospital did a midwife come to visit you?

Yes [1] → (a)
No [2] → Q46

Please do not write in this column

62

(a) How soon after you left hospital did she come?

Same day [1]
Next day [2]
Two or more days later [3]

63

46. Were you given a free gift pack or bounty bag containing things for the baby?

Yes [1] → (a)
No [2] → Q47

64

(a) Was there any baby food or drink in it?

No food or drink [1]
Yes - tick and give details [2]

65/66

47. After your baby was born were you given any free books or pamphlets which included information about feeding babies (either in a gift pack or separately)?

Yes [1]
No [2]

67

48. Since your baby was born has a health visitor been to see you?

Yes [1]
No [2]

68

(a) How old was your baby when the health visitor first came?

[ ] days old

69/70
END 03

16

START 04
SERNO=3-6
7

49. Have you taken your baby to a baby clinic yet?

Yes [1]
No [2]

50. Since the baby's birth have you been in touch with a voluntary organisation which helps new mothers (such as the National Childbirth Trust, La Leche League or the Association of Breast Feeding Mothers)?

Yes [1]
No [2]

8

51. Since you left hospital have you had any problems with feeding your baby?

(If your baby was born at home please answer about any feeding problems since the birth)

Yes [1] → (a)
No [2] → Q53

9

(a) What problems have you had? (Please describe)

MC=4
10-17

52. Did anyone give you any help or advice about this/these problems?

Yes [1] → (a)
No [2] → Q53

18

(a) Who helped or advised you?

Midwife or nurse [1]
Health visitor [2]
Doctor [3]
Friend or relative [4]
Someone else (please tick and write in) [5]

MC=4
19-22

17

70

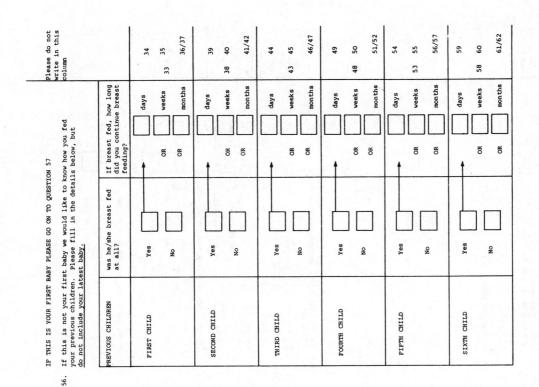

IF THIS IS YOUR FIRST BABY PLEASE GO ON TO QUESTION 57

56. If this is not your first baby we would like to know how you fed your previous children. Please fill in the details below, but do not include your latest baby.

PREVIOUS CHILDREN	was he/she breast fed at all?	If breast fed, how long did you continue breast feeding?	Please do not write in this column
FIRST CHILD	Yes ☐ No ☐	☐ days OR ☐ weeks OR ☐ months	33 34 35 36/37
SECOND CHILD	Yes ☐ No ☐	☐ days OR ☐ weeks OR ☐ months	38 39 40 41/42
THIRD CHILD	Yes ☐ No ☐	☐ days OR ☐ weeks OR ☐ months	43 44 45 46/47
FOURTH CHILD	Yes ☐ No ☐	☐ days OR ☐ weeks OR ☐ months	48 49 50 51/52
FIFTH CHILD	Yes ☐ No ☐	☐ days OR ☐ weeks OR ☐ months	53 54 55 56/57
SIXTH CHILD	Yes ☐ No ☐	☐ days OR ☐ weeks OR ☐ months	58 59 60 61/62

19

---

53. Have you ever smoked cigarettes?

   Yes ☐1 (a)
   No ☐2 Q55

Please do not write in this column — 23

(a) Do you smoke at all nowadays?

   Yes ☐1 Q54
   No ☐2 (b)

24

(b) Have you smoked at all in the past two years?

   Yes ☐1 Q54
   No ☐2 Q55

25

PLEASE WRITE IN NUMBER OF CIGARETTES A DAY
(If none write 0)

54. (a) About how many cigarettes a day were you smoking just before you became pregnant? ☐ 26/27

(b) About how many cigarettes a day were you smoking while you were pregnant? ☐ 28/29

(c) About how many cigarettes a day are you smoking now? ☐ 30/31

IF THE NUMBER SMOKED VARIES PLEASE GIVE AN AVERAGE

55. For most people having a new baby means a lot of extra expense and some people find it difficult to manage.

Thinking about how you (and your family) are managing on your money at the moment, would you say you are .....

   managing quite well ☐1
   just getting by ☐2
   or getting into difficulties? ☐3
   Other answer (Please tick and write in) ☐4

32

18

71

Finally a few questions about yourself which will help us show the kind of people the survey represents

Please do not write in this column

57.   What is your present age?

    Under 20   □ 1

    20, up to 24   □ 2

    25, up to 29   □ 3

    30 or over   □ 4

63

58.   How old were you when you finished full-time education? (School or college whichever you last attended full time)

    16 or under   □ 1

    17   □ 2

    18   □ 3

    19 or over   □ 4

64

59.   Are you doing any paid work at the moment?

    Yes   □ 1

    On paid maternity leave   □ 2 → Q60

    On unpaid maternity leave   □ 3

    No   □ 4 → (a)

65

(a)   Do you plan to start work again within the next two years?

    Yes, full time   □ 1

    Yes, part time   □ 2

    No   □ 3

    Do not know   □ 4

66

Now go to Question 61

20

Please do not write in this column

60   (a)   What is your job?
    (Please write in your job title)

67/68

(b)   What do you actually do?

(c)   What does the firm or organisation you work for make or do?

(d)   Are you .....

    an employee   □ 1 → (e)

    or self-employed   □ 2 → (f)

(e)   Are you a manager or supervisor of any kind?

    Yes, Manager   □ 1

    Yes, supervisor   □ 2

    No, neither   □ 3

(f)   Do you work mainly at home or do you go out to work?

    Mainly at home   □ 1

    Go out to work   □ 2

69

21

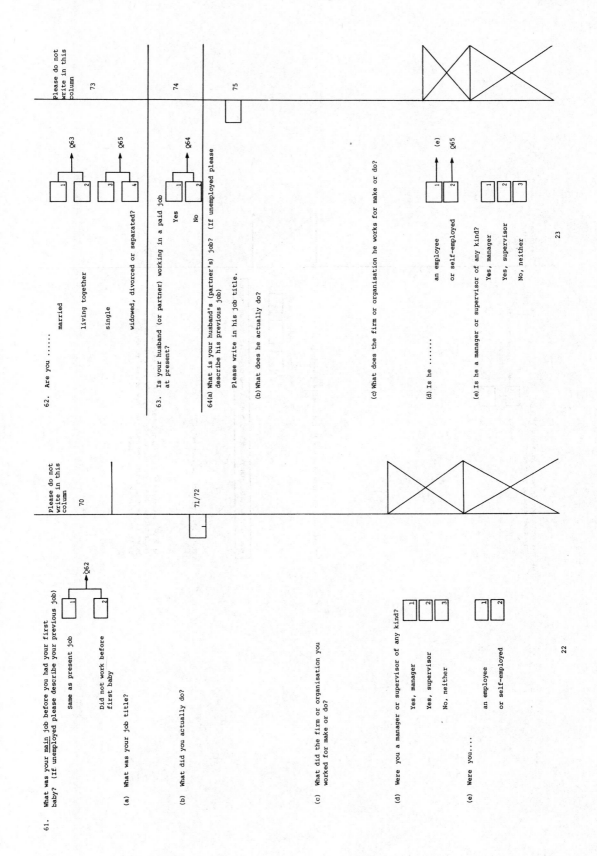

61. What was your <u>main</u> job before you had your first baby? (If unemployed please describe your previous job)

Same as present job [1] → Q62

Did not work before first baby [2]

(a) What was your job title?

(b) What did you actually do?

(c) What did the firm or organisation you worked for make or do?

(d) Were you a manager or supervisor of any kind?

Yes, manager [1]

Yes, supervisor [2]

No, neither [3]

(e) Were you....

an employee [1]

or self-employed [2]

Please do not write in this column

70

71/72

22

Please do not write in this column

73

74

75

62. Are you ......

married [1] → Q63

living together [2]

single [3] → Q65

widowed, divorced or separated [4]

63. Is your husband (or partner) working in a paid job at present?

Yes [1] → Q64

No [2]

64(a) What is your husband's (partner's) job? (If unemployed please describe his previous job)

Please write in his job title.

(b) What does he actually do?

(c) What does the firm or organisation he works for make or do?

(d) Is he ....

an employee [1]

or self-employed [2] → Q65

(e) Is he a manager or supervisor of any kind?

Yes, manager [1]

Yes, supervisor [2]

No, neither [3]

23

65. Is there anything else you would like to say about feeding your baby?

Yes ☐ 1 → please write in below

No ☐ 2

Please give the date when you filled in this questionnaire

day month year

☐ ☐ ☐ 19

WAS THERE ANYTHING YOU INTENDED TO GO BACK AND COMPLETE?   PLEASE CHECK.

Thank you very much for your help.

We hope to contact mothers again later to see how they are feeding their babies when they are a little older. If you expect to move house in the near future and know your new address it would help us if you could write it below:

24

(b) Stage 2 documents: initial letter and questionnaire

Office of Population Censuses and Surveys
Social Survey Division

St Catherines House 10 Kingsway London WC2B 6JP

Telephone 01-242 0262 ext 2256

Your reference

Our reference
S1233/E2/1

Date

January/February 1986

Dear Madam

SURVEY OF INFANT FEEDING

We contacted you several months ago asking for your help with a study of Infant Feeding which is being carried out for the Department of Health and Social Security. On that occasion you kindly completed our questionnaire and I am now writing to ask if you would help us again.

We are interested in finding out how the pattern of feeding changes as babies get older and I am enclosing a questionnaire about this which can be returned in the reply paid envelope provided.

If, for any reason, your baby is no longer with you please tick the box on the front page of the questionnaire and return it to us so that we do not trouble you further.

As in all our surveys we rely on people's voluntary cooperation. The information that you give is treated in strict confidence by OPCS. it is not released to any other Government department in any way in which it can be associated with your name or address. In published reports the identity of an individual is never revealed: the results of the survey are shown as statistics only.

Thank you in advance for your help.

Yours faithfully

Lizanne Dowds

Lizanne Dowds
Research Officer

S1233/21

01 = 1/2
SERNO = 3-6
SAMPNO = 7-15

SURVEY OF INFANT FEEDING

1 Most questions on the following pages can be answered simply by
putting a tick in the box next to the answer that applies to you.

Example: Yes [✓]₁

             No   [ ]₂

Sometimes you are asked to write in a number or the answer in your own
words. Please enter numbers as figures rather than words.

2 Usually after answering each question you go on to the next unless a
box you have ticked has an arrow next to it with an instruction to go
to another question.

Example: Yes [✓]₁ ──→ Q5

             No   [ ]₂

By following the arrows carefully you will miss out some questions which
do not apply to you, so the amount you have to fill in will make the
questionnaire shorter than it looks.

3 If you cannot remember, do not know or are unable to answer a
particular question please write that in.

4 If, rather than a single baby you have twins or triplets, please answer
the questions in relation to the one who was born first.

5 When you have finished please post the questionnaire to us as soon as
possible in the reply paid envelope provided, even if you were not
able to answer all of it.

The names and addresses of people who co-operate in our surveys are
held in strict confidence by OPCS and never passed to any other
Government Department, or to members of the public or press.

We shall be very grateful for your help.

If for any reason your baby is not with you at the moment please tick
the box below and return the questionnaire to us so we do not trouble
you further.

        My baby is no longer with me [ ]

1

1 How old is your baby?

PLEASE ENTER NUMBERS IN BOTH BOXES

Weeks ☐ and days ☐

Please do not write in this column

16-18

2 Are you still breast feeding him/her at all?

Yes ☐1 → a)

No ☐2 → Q3

19

a) Do you give him/her milk from a bottle at present (apart from expressed breast milk)?

Yes ☐1 → Q4

No ☐2 → Q9

20

3 How old was your baby when you last breast fed him/her?

PLEASE ENTER NUMBERS IN BOTH BOXES

Weeks ☐ and days ☐

21-23

b) What were your reasons for stopping breast feeding? (Please explain all your reasons)

MC=5

24-33

2

---

4 Which kind of milk do you give your baby at the moment?

	Cow and Gate Premium	☐	01
	Cow and Gate Plus	☐	02
PLEASE	Cow and Gate Formula S	☐	03
TICK	SMA Gold Cap	☐	07
ONE BOX	SMA White Cap	☐	08
ONLY	Wysoy	☐	09
	Milupa Milumil	☐	10
	Milupa Aptamil	☐	11
	Progress	☐	12
	Liquid cow's milk – whole	☐	13
	– semi-skimmed	☐	14
	– skimmed	☐	15
	Another kind of milk (please tick and write in the name)	☐	16

Please do not write in this column

34/35

[NOTE: Osterfeed and Ostermilk have been temporarily withdrawn]

5. How old was your baby when you started giving this kind of milk?

PLEASE ENTER A NUMBER IN THE BOX

Weeks ☐

36-45

3

6 The labels on tins or packets of baby milk tell you about the contents of the milk. Do you read this information?

Yes – usually   [1] ⎤
Yes – sometimes [2] ⎦ → a) – c)
No – never [3] → Q7

46

a) How easy do you find it to understand this information?

very easy [1]
Quite easy [2]
Quite difficult [3]
Very difficult [4]

47

b) Do you find the information helpful?

Yes [1]
No [2]

48

c) What changes in the information about the content of baby milk would you like to see on the label?

None – I am satisfied with what is said on the label [1]

The same information but explained more clearly [2]

The exact quantities of each ingredient [3]

Something else (please tick and write in) [4]

MC = 4

49-52

4

---

7 Apart from the contents of the milk what additional information would you like to see on the label?

MC = 4

53-60

8 About how much a week do you spend on milk for your baby?

PLEASE ENTER NUMBERS IN BOTH BOXES

pounds   and   pence

61-64

9 Do you get milk tokens?

Yes – for the baby [1]
Yes – for myself [2]
Yes – for older child [3]
Have applied for tokens [4]
No – I don't get tokens [5]

MC = 3

65-67

10 Now a few questions on solid foods.

Do you give your baby foods such as cereal, rusks or any other kind of solid food including any that you make yourself?

Yes [1] → a)
No [2] → Q16

68

a) How old was your baby when he/she first had any food apart from milk?

PLEASE ENTER A NUMBER IN THE BOX

Weeks

69/70

End 01

5

a) How easy do you find it to understand this information?

- Very easy [1]
- Quite easy [2]
- Quite difficult [3]
- Very difficult [4]

25

b) Do you find the information helpful?

- Yes [1]
- No [2]

26

c) What changes in the information about the content of baby food would you like to see on the label?

- None – I am satisfied with what is said on the label [1]
- The same information but explained more clearly [2]
- The exact quantities of each ingredient [3]
- Something else (please tick and write in) [4]

MC=4
27-30

14 a) Apart from the contents of the food what additional information would you like to see on the label?

MC=4
31-38

14 b) What do you take into account when deciding what solid foods to give your baby?

MC=5
39-48

7

Start 02
SERNO=3-6

11 Thinking back to yesterday, can you list all the cereal, rusks or solid food that your baby ate. Please describe each fully, giving the brand name or if its home made, whether the food is stage 1 or 2 (or infant or junior) and also the time of the feed.

Didn't have solids yesterday [1] → Q12

7

Time of feed	Type of food and stage	Brand (or Home made)

MC=7
8-21

12 Do you use milk to mix up your baby's food?

- Yes [1] → a)
- No [2]

22

a) Do you use

- infant formula milk [1]
- or liquid cow's milk [2]
- or something else (please tick and write in) [3]

23

13 The labels on tins or packets of baby food tell you about the contents of the food. Do you read this information?

- Yes – usually [1] → a) - c)
- Yes – sometimes [2]
- No – never [3] → Q14

24

6

Page 8

15   About how much a week do you spend on solid food
     for the baby (including any you make yourself)?

     PLEASE ENTER NUMBERS IN BOXES
     Pounds   Pence
     [ ]   and   [ ]

16   Apart from milk do you give your baby water or anything
     else to drink?

     Yes [1] → a)
     No [2] → Q19

a)   Please tick boxes and/or write in the drink your baby
     usually has. Please give the brand name, flavour and
     say if it is a special baby drink or not.

     Plain water   [1]
     Water with sugar
     or honey added   [2]

Brand name	Flavour	Please tick if it is a baby drink

8

Page 9

17   Do you give your baby drinks mainly .....

     because he/she is thirsty   [1]
     to give him/her extra vitamins   [2]
     to help his/her digestion   [3]
     or for some other reason
     (please tick and write in)   [4]

18   About how much a week do you spend on drinks for your
     baby?

     PLEASE ENTER NUMBERS IN BOXES

     Pounds   Pence
     [ ]   and   [ ]

19   Do you give your baby any extra vitamins (apart from
     vitamin drinks mentioned at Q16)?

     Yes [1] → a) & b)
     No [2] → Q20

a)   Do you use Childrens Vitamin Drops from the clinic
     or another brand?

     Childrens Vitamin Drops   [1]
     Other brand (please tick and
     write in full name)   [2]

b)   How do you get the vitamins?

     Buy the vitamins myself   [1]
     Get vitamins free at the clinic   [2]
     Get vitamins on prescription   [3]
     Other (please tick and write in)   [4]

9

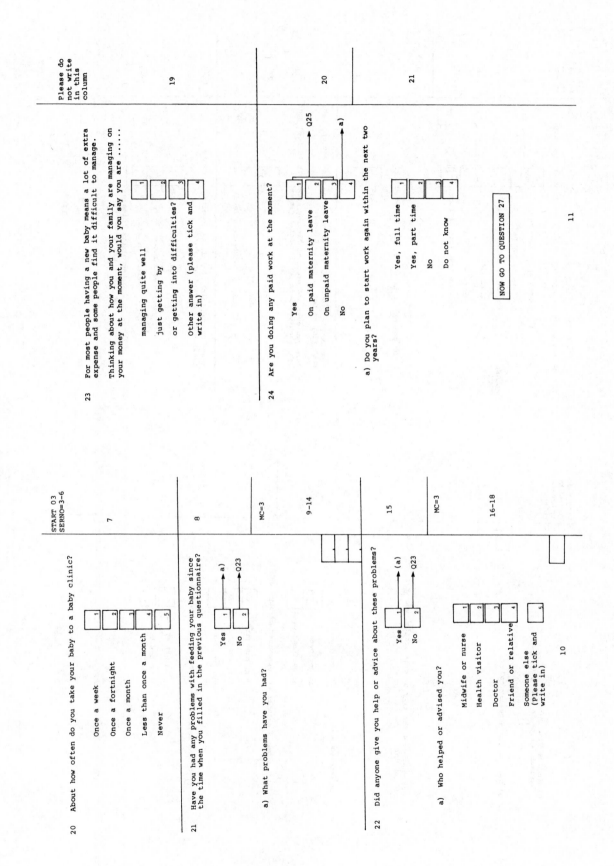

20. About how often do you take your baby to a baby clinic?

- Once a week [1]
- Once a fortnight [2]
- Once a month [3]
- Less than once a month [4]
- Never [5]

START 03
SERNO=3-6

7

21. Have you had any problems with feeding your baby since the time when you filled in the previous questionnaire?

- Yes [1] → a)
- No [2] → Q23

8

a) What problems have you had?

MC=3

9-14

22. Did anyone give you help or advice about these problems?

- Yes [1] → (a)
- No [2] → Q23

15

a) Who helped or advised you?

- Midwife or nurse [1]
- Health visitor [2]
- Doctor [3]
- Friend or relative [4]
- Someone else (Please tick and write in) [5]

MC=3

16-18

10

23. For most people having a new baby means a lot of extra expense and some people find it difficult to manage.

Thinking about how you and your family are managing on your money at the moment, would you say you are ......

- managing quite well [1]
- just getting by [2]
- or getting into difficulties? [3]
- Other answer (please tick and write in) [4]

Please do not write in this column

19

24. Are you doing any paid work at the moment?

Yes
- On paid maternity leave [1]
- On unpaid maternity leave [2]
- No [3]

[1][2][3] → Q25
[4] → a)

20

a) Do you plan to start work again within the next two years?

- Yes, full time [1]
- Yes, part time [2]
- No [3]
- Do not know [4]

21

NOW GO TO QUESTION 27

11

25 a) What is your job? (Please write in your job title)

b) What do you actually do?

c) What does the firm or organisation you work for make or do?

d) Are you ....

an employee [1]

or self-employed [2]

e) Are you a manager or supervisor of any kind?

Yes, manager [1]

Yes, supervisor [2]

No, neither [3]

f) Do you work mainly at home or do you go out to work?

Mainly at home [1]

Go out to work [2]

24

12

---

26 When you are working who usually looks after the baby?

PLEASE TICK ONE ONLY

No-one apart from me [1] → Q27

Husband or partner [2]

Mother or mother-in-law [3]

Childminder [4] → a)

Nursery or crèche [5]

Someone else (please tick and write in) [6]

25

a) Do you pay to have the baby looked after?

Yes [1]

No [2]

26

27 Some people find it difficult to manage with a young baby when they go out to public places.

Have you ever had problems finding somewhere to feed your baby when you were out in public places?

Yes [1]

No [2]

Only go out between feeds [3]

27

28 Where do you think that it is important to have facilities for feeding babies?

shops/shopping centres [1]

restaurants [2]

public toilets [3]

Other places (please tick and write in) [4]

MC=4

28-31

13

Please give the date when you filled in this questionnaire

day month Year

19

WAS THERE ANYTHING YOU INTENDED TO GO BACK AND COMPLETE?

PLEASE CHECK

Thank you very much for your help.

We hope to contact mothers again later on to see how they are feeding their babies when they are a little older. If you expect to move house in the near future and know your new address it would help us if you could write it below:

15

Please do not write in this column

29 Have you ever had problems finding somewhere to change your baby when you were out in public places?

Yes 1
No 2
Don't change the baby when I'm out 3

32

30 Where do you think it is important to have facilities for changing babies?

shops/shopping centres 1
restaurants 2
public toilets 3
Other places (please tick and write in) 4

MC=4

33-36

31 Is there anything else you would like to say about feeding your baby?

Yes 1
No 2

Please write in below

37

14

(c) Stage 3 documents: initial letter and questionnaire

Office of Population Censuses and Surveys
Social Survey Division
St Catherines House 10 Kingsway London WC2B 6JP
Telephone 01-242 0262 ext 2256

Your reference

Our reference
S1233/E3/1

Date

June 1986

Dear Madam

SURVEY OF INFANT FEEDING

We contacted you twice over the last 9 months asking for your help with a study of
Infant Feeding which is being carried out for the Department of Health and Social
Security. On both occasions you kindly completed our questionnaire and I am now
writing to ask if you will help us with the final stage of the survey.

We are interested in how the pattern of feeding changes as babies reach 9 to 10 months
and I am enclosing a questionnaire about this which can be returned in the reply
paid envelope provided.

If, for any reason, your baby is no longer with you please tick the box on the front
page of the questionnaire and return it to us so that we do not trouble you further.

As in all our surveys we rely on people's voluntary cooperation. The information
that you give is treated in strict confidence by OPCS. It is not released to any
other Government Department in any way in which it can be associated with your name
or address. No information about you as an individual or your particular household
is ever passed to members of the public or the press. The published reports contain
no information about individual people; the results of the survey are shown as
statistics only.

Thank you in advance for your help.

Yours faithfully

Lizanne Dowds

Lizanne Dowds
Research Officer

S1233/31

01=1/2
SERNO=3-6
SAMPNO=7-15
☐☐

SURVEY OF INFANT FEEDING

1 Most questions on the following pages can be answered simply by putting a tick in the box next to the answer that applies to you.

Example:

Yes ☑ 1

No ☐ 2

Sometimes you are asked to write in a number or the answer in your own words. Please enter numbers as figures rather than words.

2 Usually after answering each question you go on to the next unless a box you have ticked has an arrow next to it with an instruction to go to another question.

Example:

Yes ☑ 1 → Q5

No ☐ 2

By following the arrows carefully you will miss out some questions which do not apply to you, so the amount you have to fill in will make the questionnaire shorter than it looks.

3 If you cannot remember, do not know or are unable to answer a particular question please write that in.

4 If, rather than a single baby you had twins or triplets, please answer the questions in relation to the one who was born first.

5 When you have finished please post the questionnaire to us as soon as possible in the reply paid envelope provided, even if you were not able to answer all of it.

The information that you give is treated in strict confidence by OPCS. It is not released to other Government departments in any way in which it can be associated with your name or address. No information about you as an individual or your particular household is ever passed to members of the public or the press.

We shall be very grateful for your help.

If for any reason your baby is not with you at the moment please tick the box below and return the questionnaire to us so that we do not trouble you further.

My baby is not with me ☐

85

1 How old is your baby?

PLEASE ENTER NUMBERS IN BOTH BOXES

Weeks [ ] and [ ] days   16-18

2 Are you still breast feeding him/her at all?

Yes [1] → a)
No [2] → Q3   19

a) Do you give him/her milk from a bottle or cup at present (apart from expressed breast milk)?

Yes from a bottle or cup [1] → Q4
No [2] → Q6   20

3 How old was your baby when you last breast fed him/her?

PLEASE ENTER NUMBERS IN BOTH BOXES

Weeks [ ] and [ ] days   21-23

a) What were your reasons for stopping breast feeding? (please explain all your reasons)   MC=5 24-33

[ ][ ][ ][ ][ ]

---

4 Which kinds of milk do you give your baby to drink at the moment (apart from breastmilk)?

	Usual milk	Other milk
Cow and Gate Premium	01	01
Cow and Gate Plus	02	02
Cow and Gate Formula S	03	03
SMA Gold Cap	07	07
SMA White Cap	08	08
Wysoy	09	09
Milupa Milumil	10	10
Milupa Aptamil	11	11
Progress	12	12
Liquid cow's milk – whole	13	13
– semi-skimmed	14	14
– skimmed	15	15
Another kind of milk (Please tick and write in the name)	16	16

34-35
36-37
[ ][ ]

a) How old was your baby when you started giving each kind of milk?

Usual milk   Other milk
Weeks [ ]   weeks [ ]
Gave from birth [ ]   Gave from birth [ ]   38-41

b) About how much of each of these milks did your baby have yesterday?

Usual milk   Other milk
Fluid ozs or Mls [ ]   Fluid ozs or Mls [ ]   42-45

86

5 About how much a week do you spend on milk for your baby?

PLEASE ENTER NUMBERS IN THE BOXES

pounds [ ] and pence [ ]

46-49

6 Do you get milk tokens?

Yes - for the baby [1]
Yes - for myself [2]
Yes - for older child [3]
Have applied for tokens [4]
No I don't get tokens [5]

MC=3

7 Apart from milk do you give your baby water or anything else to drink?

Yes [1] → a)
No [2] → Q9

50-52

a) Please tick boxes and/or write in the drink your baby usually has. Please give the brand name, flavour and say if it is a special baby drink or not.

Plain water [1]
Water with sugar or honey added [2]

53

Brand name	Flavour	Please tick if it is a baby drink

54

55-64

MC=5

8 About how much a week do you spend on drinks for your baby?

PLEASE ENTER NUMBERS IN THE BOXES

Pounds [ ] and Pence [ ]

65-68

9 Do you give your baby any extra vitamins (apart from vitamin drinks mentioned at Q7)?

Yes [1] → a) & b)
No [2] → Q10

69

a) Do you use Childrens Vitamin Drops from the clinic or another brand?

Childrens Vitamin Drops [1]
Other brand (please tick and write in full name) [2]

70

b) How do you get the vitamins?

Buy the vitamins myself at the clinic [1]
Buy the vitamins myself somewhere else [2]
Get vitamins free at the clinic [3]
Get vitamins on prescription [4]
Other (please tick and write in) [5]

71

10 Now a few questions on solid foods.

Do you give your baby foods such as cereal, rusks or any other kind of solid food including any that you make yourself?

Yes [1] → a)
No [2] → Q19

72

a) How old was your baby when he/she first had any food apart from milk?

PLEASE ENTER A NUMBER IN THE BOX

[ ] weeks

73/74
END 01

11 Have you ever used liquid cow's milk for mixing solid foods?

Yes →a) ☐1
No →Q12 ☐2

a) How old was your baby when you first gave him/her liquid cow's milk in this way?

PLEASE ENTER A NUMBER IN THE BOX

☐ weeks

7 | Start 02 SERN03–6

8/9

12 Thinking back to yesterday, can you list all the cereal, rusks or solid food that your baby ate. Please describe each fully, giving the brand name or if its homemade, whether the food is stage 1 or 2 (or infant or junior) and also the time of the meal.

Didn't have solids yesterday ☐1 →Q13

Time of Day	Type of food and stage	Brand (or homemade)

MC=7

11–24

13 About how much a week do you spend on solid food for the baby (including any you make yourself)?

PLEASE ENTER NUMBERS IN THE BOXES

Pounds ☐ and Pence ☐

25–28

---

14 The labels on tins or packets of baby food tell you about the contents of the food. Do you read this information?

Yes – usually   ☐1 ⎤
Yes – sometimes ☐2 ⎦ →a) – c)
No – never   ☐3 →Q15
Don't buy tins or packets of baby food ☐4 →Q16

29

a) How easy do you find it to understand this information?

Very easy   ☐1
Quite easy   ☐2
Quite difficult ☐3
Very difficult ☐4

30

b) Do you find the information helpful?

Yes ☐1
No ☐2

31

c) What changes in the information about the content of baby food would you like to see on the label?

None – I am satisfied with what is said on the label ☐1

The same information but explained more clearly ☐2

The exact quantities of each ingredient ☐3

Something else (please tick and write in) ☐4

MC=4

32–35

☐

88

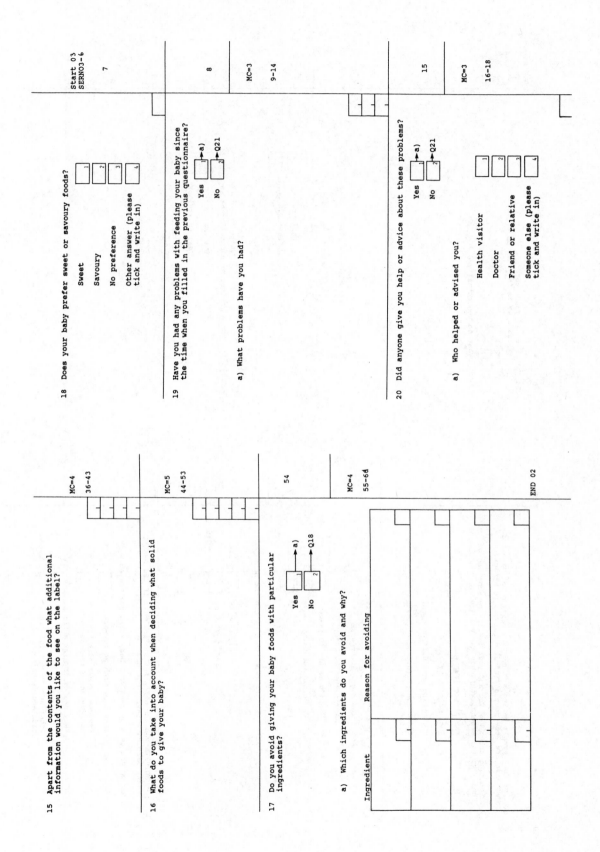

15 Apart from the contents of the food what additional information would you like to see on the label?

MC=4
36-43

16 What do you take into account when deciding what solid foods to give your baby?

MC=5
44-53

17 Do you avoid giving your baby foods with particular ingredients?

Yes 1 → a)
No 2 → Q18

54

a) Which ingredients do you avoid and why?

Ingredient   Reason for avoiding

MC=4
55-6d

END 02

18 Does your baby prefer sweet or savoury foods?

Sweet 1
Savoury 2
No preference 3
Other answer (please tick and write in) 4

Start 03
SERNO3-6
7

19 Have you had any problems with feeding your baby since the time when you filled in the previous questionnaire?

Yes 1 → a)
No 2 → Q21

8

a) What problems have you had?

MC=3
9-14

20 Did anyone give you help or advice about these problems?

Yes 1 → a)
No 2 → Q21

15

a) Who helped or advised you?

Health visitor 1
Doctor 2
Friend or relative 3
Someone else (please tick and write in) 4

MC=3
16-18

24 a) What is your job?
(Please write in your job title)

25/26

b) What do you actually do?

c) What does the firm or organisation you work for make or do?

d) Are you....

an employee ☐
or self-employed ☐

e) Are you a manager or supervisor of any kind?

Yes, manager ☐
Yes, supervisor ☐
No, neither ☐

---

21 For most people having a young baby means a lot of extra expense and some people find it difficult to manage.

Thinking about how you and your family are managing on your money at the moment, would you say you are....

managing quite well [1]
just getting by [2]
or getting into difficulties? [3]
Other answer (please tick and write in) [4]

19

22 Are you doing any paid work at the moment?

Yes - go out to work → Q23
Yes - work at home → Q24
On paid maternity leave
On unpaid maternity leave
No → a)

20

a) Do you plan to start work again within the next two years?

Yes, full time
Yes, part time
No → Q26
Don't know

21

23 FOR MOTHERS WHO ARE STILL BREAST FEEDING. IF YOU ARE NOT BREAST FEEDING PLEASE GO TO Q24

MC=3

How do you usually feed your baby while you are at work?

Take baby with me to work [1]
Express breast milk for baby to have while I am at work [2]
Baby has other milk while I am at work [3]
Other arrangement (please tick and describe [4]

22-24

25 When you are working who usually looks after the baby?

PLEASE TICK
ONE ONLY

No-one apart from me □1 → Q26

Husband or partner □2

Mother or mother-in-law □3 → a)

Childminder □4

Nursery or creche □5

Someone else (please tick and write in) □6

27

a) Do you pay to have the baby looked after?

Yes □1

No □2

28

26 When you look back on how you have fed your baby since his/her birth are you happy with everything you decided to do or do you wish that you had made other decisions about how to feed him/her?

I am happy with my decisions □1 → Q27

I wish I had made other decisions □2 → a)

29

a) Looking back, what decisions would you have made?

MC=3

30-32

27 Is there anything else you would like to say about feeding your baby?

Yes □1 Please write in below

No □2

Please give the date when you filled in this questionnaire

day □ month □ year □

┌───┐
│ WAS THERE ANYTHING YOU INTENDED TO GO BACK AND COMPLETE? │
│ PLEASE CHECK │
└───┘

Thank you very much for your help.

Printed in the United Kingdom for Her Majesty's Stationery Office
Dd290875 C10 5/88 0443/5 59471

WEST HERTFORDSHIRE
SCHOOL OF MIDWIFERY